NEW REPRODUCTIVE TECHNOLOGIES
AND DISEMBODIMENT

For Heather,
with all my love (+ gratitude)
always,
Paula.

Theory, Technology and Society

Series Editor: Ross Abbinnett, University of Birmingham, UK

Theory, Technology and Society presents the latest work in social, cultural and political theory, which considers the impact of new technologies on social, economic and political relationships. Central to the series are the elucidation of new theories of the humanity-technology relationship, the ethical implications of techno-scientific innovation, and the identification of unforeseen effects which are emerging from the techno-scientific organization of society.

With particular interest in questions of gender relations, the body, virtuality, penality, work, aesthetics, urban space, surveillance, governance and the environment, the series encourages work that seeks to determine the nature of the social consequences that have followed the deployment of new technologies, investigate the increasingly complex relationship between 'the human' and 'the technological', or addresses the ethical and political questions arising from the constant transformation and manipulation of humanity.

Other titles in this series

Urban Constellations
Spaces of Cultural Regeneration in Post-Industrial Britain
Zoë Thompson
ISBN 978 1 4724 2722 9

Eventful Bodies
The Cosmopolitics of Illness
Michael Schillmeier
ISBN 978 1 4094 4982 9

Genetics as Social Practice
Transdisciplinary Views on Science and Culture
Edited by Barbara Prainsack, Silke Schicktanz, Gabriele Werner-Felmayer
ISBN 978 1 4094 5548 6

The Visualised Foetus
A Cultural and Political Analysis of Ultrasound Imagery
Julie Roberts
ISBN 978 1 4094 2939 5

New Reproductive Technologies and Disembodiment

Feminist and Material Resolutions

CARLA LAM
University of Otago, New Zealand

ASHGATE

Published by
Ashgate Publishing Limited
Wey Court East
Union Road
Farnham
Surrey, GU9 7PT
England

Ashgate Publishing Company
110 Cherry Street
Suite 3-1
Burlington, VT 05401-3818
USA

www.ashgate.com

British Library Cataloguing in Publication Data
A catalogue record for this book is available from the British Library

The Library of Congress has cataloged the printed edition as follows:
Lam, Carla.
   New reproductive technologies and disembodiment : feminist and material resolutions / by Carla Lam.
      pages cm. – (Theory, technology and society)
   Includes bibliographical references and index.
   ISBN 978-1-4724-3705-1 (hardback) – ISBN 978-1-4724-3706-8 (ebook) –
   ISBN 978-1-4724-3707-5 (epub) 1. Human reproductive technology–Social aspects.
2. Human reproduction–Social aspects. 3. Women–Psychology. 4. Feminist theory.
I. Title.

   GN482.1.L36 2014
   305.4201--dc23

                                                                                        2014033842

ISBN 9781472437051 (hbk)
ISBN 9781472437068 (ebk – PDF)
ISBN 9781472437075 (ebk – ePUB)

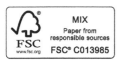

Printed in the United Kingdom by Henry Ling Limited,
at the Dorset Press, Dorchester, DT1 1HD

Contents

Acknowledgements   *vii*

Introduction: Disembodiment   1

PART I: REPRODUCTION IN THE TWENTY-FIRST CENTURY

1   New Reproductive Technologies and Disembodiment   21

PART II: FEMINISM AND NEW REPRODUCTIVE TECHNOLOGIES

2   Resistors and Embracers   41

3   Equivocals   65

PART III: MATERIAL RESOLUTIONS

4   Mary O'Brien and 'The Feminist Standpoint Revisited'   81

5   Postconstructionist, 'New' Material Feminisms: Breaking
     Feminist Waves   97

Conclusion   117

Bibliography   *131*
Index   *153*

Acknowledgements

This book was born of an enormous and long-term effort supported by many people, and the University of Otago through my department of politics there. I have due gratitude for the Performance Based Research Fund at the University of Otago, and the human translation into a series of research assistants, including Iona Mylek, Emma King, and most recently, Stevie Jepson for crucial support. Without the understanding of my students and tutors including especially Lynne Bowyer, the journey to completion would have been significantly increased – especially at the end.

I am indebted to my colleagues at the politics department for various forms of support and care, but especially to Lena Tan and Janine Hayward. A special thank you also to Robert Patman whose dogged, stalwart belief in the project and its completion arrived when any other response would have signalled its death knell. Furthermore, the mentoring friendship and support of Heather Devere and Jay Smith was significant in bringing this book to light – thank you.

I am perpetually thankful for my sister, mother and father, friends near and far especially Lindsey McKay who has shared all aspects of this process with me over the years. Special recognition also goes to Lena Tan (a dear friend as well as a colleague since I arrived in New Zealand) and Sarah Lovell for moral support, pep talks and unfailingly excellent advice. Finally, thank you to Ashgate whose helpful reviews, editor and administrator made the process easy.

Introduction
Disembodiment

In the early twenty-first century, new reproductive technologies (NRTs) facilitate the literal disembodiment of reproduction. *In vitro* fertilization (IVF), embryo transfer (ET), and cloning take conception outside the female body; development of an artificial womb promises to take gestation outside the uterus; and practices such as pre-scheduled caesarean sections (C-Sections) ensure that birth itself will be technologically mediated and a medical process that largely takes place outside of the mother's body. Furthermore, new monitoring technologies that visualize and test the unborn foetus allow for greater medicalization of both pregnancy and birth. These may give women a greater sense of security and control, but they can also restrict their embodied knowledge and experiences. Similarly, surrogacy disaggregates reproduction and redefines motherhood, and biology itself, reimagining and transforming the reproductive process into a series of commodifiable, discrete transactions. This technological mediation, in and of itself, is not unwelcome; however, it potentially represses less technological models and opens up women's bodies to control by patriarchal and capitalist interests.[1] Interests which often support the marketization of social services (including medicine), a rise in health 'sciences' (over healthcare), trans-local communications networks, and a political climate defined by neoliberalism, post-feminism and a general decline in identity politics. As such, NRTs are part of the biotech 'revolution' of postmodernity, and the accelerated 'geneticization' of contemporary life.[2]

Discourse surrounding biotechnology conforms to polarized theorizations that amount to restatements of the biology/society debate. This book uniquely

---

1 Robbie E. Davis-Floyd, 'The Technocratic Body and the Organic Body: Cultural Models for Women's Birth Choices', in *Knowledge and Society: The Anthology of Science and Technology*, Vol. 9, ed. David Hess and Linda Layen, Greenwich, CT: JAI Press Inc., 1992, 59–93.

2 Brewster Kneen, *Farmageddon: Food and the Culture of Biotechnology*, Gabriola Island, BC: New Society Publishers, 1999; Radha Holla-Bhar and Vandana Shiva, 'Piracy by Patent: The Case of the Neem Tree', in *The Case Against the Global Economy And For a Turn Toward the Local*, ed. Jerry Mander and Edward Goldsmith, San Francisco: Sierra Club Books, 1996, 146–59; Andrew Kimbrell, 'Biocolonization: The Patenting of Life and the Global Market in Body Parts', in *The Case Against the Global Economy And For a Turn Toward the Local*, ed. Jerry Mander and Edward Goldsmith, San Francisco: Sierra Club Books, 1996, 131–45; Abby Lippman, 'Worrying – and Worrying About – the Geneticization of Reproduction and Health', in *Misconceptions: The Social Construction of Choice and the New Reproductive and Genetic Technologies*, Vol. 1, ed. Gwynne Basen, Margrit Eichler and Abby Lippman, Quebec: Voyageur Publishing, 1993, 39–65.

emphasizes the continuing importance of this debate as underpinning many current issues including, but not limited to, biotechnology. This Western dualism goes back at least as far as the ancient Greek thought of Plato and continues to emerge in both orthodox and much critical (including feminist) political theory today. My approach ultimately attempts to mitigate this polarization and its effects by complicating the over-simple, and longstanding dualistic patterns of thought on which the biology/society oppositional pairing is based. This is not a new endeavour in feminist theory and focuses on the biosocial approach to embodiment (and identity) as constructed through the work of scholars in the tradition of Ruth Hubbard, Thomas Laqueur, Ann Fausto-Sterling and especially Mary O'Brien whose feminist materialist analysis comes to bear on the continuing development of reproductive technologies but has been overlooked because of its imbrication in the biological essentialist/social constructionist division within academic feminism. Such work spans disciplines, but has often been understood as feminist science and technology studies (FSTS). Furthermore, I situate my work as part of the 'post-constructionist turn' in social and political theory, that emphasizes materiality as a kind of workable settlement between biological determinism and social essentialism which both perpetuate longstanding patriarchal dualism in its various and overlapping manifestations, like mind versus body, and society versus biology.[3] This complex negotiation has inseparable methodological, ontological and epistemological consequences, or in feminist physicist Karen Barad's rather helpful term 'onto-epistemological'[4] ones that highlight 'the inseparability of being and knowing'.[5] It is as such that post-constructionist material feminisms potentially deliver on the unfulfilled claims about material agency made in good faith by both modern and postmodern epistemological traditions in feminism.[6] Barad's neologism puts into circulation more longstanding feminist epistemological thinking, as an endeavour concerned predominantly with the ethical dimensions of all ways of knowing, or knowledge as situated practice only understood in social and political contexts.

Nina Lykke's useful phrasing, 'the post-constructionist turn' refers also to 'post-constructionism' as a new methodological tool, or 'thinking technology' (from Haraway), which provides a crucial platform of exchange to discuss trans-dualistic

---

3   Nina Lykke, 'The Timeliness of Post-Constructionism', *NORA – Nordic Journal of Feminist and Gender Research* 18:2 (June 2010): 131–6.

4   Karen Barad, 'Getting Real: Technoscientific Practices and the Materialization of Reality', *Differences: A Journal of Feminist Cultural Studies* 10:2 (1998).

5   It blends feminist theory and Niels Bohr's philosophy of quantum physics and which Barad unfolds over several works. See Nina Lykke, *Feminist Studies: A Guide to Intersectional Theory, Methodology, and Writing*, New York: Routledge, 2010.

6   See for example, Lykke, 'The Timeliness of Post-Constructionism' and Iris van der Tuin and Rick Dolphijn, 'The Transversality of New Materialism', *Women: A Cultural Review* 21:2 (2010): 159.

theory developments rather than emphasizing similarities or commonalities.[7] More specifically, post-constructionism refers 'to different epistemological positions that share a commitment to a double move *into* and *beyond* postmodern philosophy and post-structuralism'.[8] Post-constructionist feminist theories are also sometimes controversially referred to as 'new material feminisms' and in this book I will use these two terms interchangeably, only adding other terms in fidelity to individual author's preferences for the same concepts.

Some feminist scholars read the new reproductive technologies as the latest chapter in the long history of the misappropriation of women's reproduction into androcentric Western understandings through techno-science, and medicine. This Western paradigm by which women's embodied power is assimilated into patriarchal culture and politics through the attribution of women's reproductive roles to men, I call *birth appropriation*. Adam creates Eve out of his body, Zeus 'gives birth' to Athena from his head, men become 'fathers' of the democracy, the nation, the church and so on. Yet new reproductive technologies reveal the paradox of women's reproductive experiences in patriarchal cultures as both, and often simultaneously, experiences of power and vulnerability.[9] I would argue that NRTs indicate a postmodern[10] instantiation of birth appropriation because they represent a new conceptual and material relationship of humans to nature that builds on, yet is distinct from, modern understandings.

In *The Politics of Reproduction*, O'Brien argues for two moments of 'world historically' significant change in birth process – the discovery of physiological paternity and the advent of mass contraceptive technology. These provided the material grounds for new configurations of the human condition at the levels of ideas and society. In the following chapters, I argue that NRTs constitute a

---

7 She writes, 'I consider 'postconstructionism' to be a temporarily useful framework for joint theoretical reflections and negotiations rather than a definition carved in stone', Lykke, *Feminist Studies*, 134.

8 Lykke, *Feminist Studies*, 209. Emphasis added.

9 See Shiloh Y. Whitney, 'Dependency Relations: Corporeal Vulnerability and Norms of Personhood in Hobbes and Kittay', *Hypatia* 26:2 (Summer 2011): 554–74.

10 The terms postmodernism and poststructuralism tend to be used interchangeably and I will do the same here. Judith Grant also conflates the two as 'ways to refer to a loosely affiliated though internally diverse body of thought that has common epistemological and ontological roots in the philosophy of Nietzsche' (*Fundamental Feminism*, London: Routledge, 1993). For my purposes, I want to explore postmodernism as a somewhat cohesive critical approach (or state of mind) to certain features of Enlightenment modernism, especially the unified subject animated by a rational, self-directed and autonomous agency. How this matters to reproduction is in how it challenges paradigms of identity politics, especially women's identity politics (or Western feminist claims) and this is my concern. The argument here is that postmodern reproductive politics differ from, and yet are coextensive with modern, Enlightenment ones – to a certain extent materially but moreover ideologically, and that this difference matters to disembodiment (both conceptual and material) for both women and men, though my focus is on women.

new material reproductive process reflected in profound, radically new social relations, and new reproductive consciousnesses: in a term, new reproductive praxis. Further, this third moment disembodies women in unprecedented ways, as evident in recent popular and academic texts, especially those associated with postmodernism. Furthermore, I take a closer look at where the sexed body has gone within feminist theory, and am concerned about the onto-epistemological implications of postmodernism for gendered subjectivity, especially in light of the disembodiment effected by new reproductive technologies.[11]

O'Brien's attribution of 'world historical' feels dramatically out of place in twenty-first-century academia, since it implies some element of universal experience in reproductive consciousness. As she explains, 'We are not at all engaged in a psychology of pregnancy, or in the subjective experience of one man who parts with his seed and one woman whose femininity involuntarily creates and gives birth to one or more children'.[12] O'Brien's argument for the universal significance of these historical changes in birth process proved contentious in 1981 when it was first published amidst critiques of second-wave feminism's projection of an overall privileged woman as its 'universal' and neutral subject. As such it bears the marks of the second- to third-wave feminist cusp with ongoing tensions still playing out in feminist debates, including those about whether recently emerging materialist theories with clear resonance in older ones, are actually meaningfully 'new'.[13]

But O'Brien's materialist theory of reproduction deserves re-examination because of its potential contribution to current reproductive politics and feminist thought. This is especially so given the growing literature on (new) material

---

11   Lykke, *Feminist Studies*; Annette Burfoot, 'In-Appropriation – A Critique of "Proceed with Care: Final Report of the Royal Commission on New Reproductive Technologies"', *Women's Studies International Forum* 18:4 (1995): 499–506.

12   Mary O'Brien, *The Politics of Reproduction*, Boston: Routledge and Kegan Paul, 1981, 50.

13   Sara Ahmed, 'Open Forum Imaginary Prohibitions: Some Preliminary Remarks on the Founding Gestures of the "New Materialism"', *European Journal of Women's Studies* 15:1 (2008): 23–39; Iris Van der Tuin, 'Deflationary Logic: Response to Sara Ahmed's "Imaginary Prohibitions: Some Preliminary Remarks on the Founding Gestures of the 'New Materialism'"', *European Journal of Women's Studies* 15:4 (2008): 411–16; Noela Davis, 'New Materialism and Feminism's Anti-Biologism: A Response to Sara Ahmed', *European Journal of Women's Studies* 16:1 (2009): 67–80; Clare Hemmings, *Why Stories Matter: The Political Grammar of Feminist Theory*, Durham: Duke University Press, 2011; Karen Barad, 'Getting Real: Technoscientific Practices and the Materialization of Reality', *Differences: A Journal of Feminist Cultural Studies* 10:2 (1998); Lynda Birke and Cecilia Asberg, 'Biology is a feminist issue: Interview with Lynda Birke', *European Journal of Women's Studies* 17:4 (2010): 413–23.; Myra J. Hird, 'Feminist Matters: New Materialist Considerations of Sexual Difference', *Feminist Theory* 5:2 (2004): 223–32; Sari Irni, 'Sex, Power and Ontology: Exploring the Performativity of Hormones', *NORA – Nordic Journal of Feminist and Gender Research* 21:1 (2013): 41–56; Lykke, *Feminist Studies*.

feminisms which reinforce and build on the biosocial notion of reproduction she asserted.[14] While the open parameters of O'Brien's theory need attention, her work highlights male and female reproductive experiences of normative and epistemological significance related to the differentiated corporeality of sex/ reproduction which NRTs erode.

Recognizing commonalities in women's experiences need not mean overriding differences. O'Brien's argument that 'there is an aspect of human understanding which might be called reproductive consciousness' that is 'differentiated by gender' does not preclude the recognition that other class memberships also differentiate reproductive consciousness.[15] Indeed, this argument explains the variety of reproductive knowledge among women. For example, an adequate reproductive dialectical materialism must take into account that poverty affects sexuality and reproduction. Most explicitly, menstruation is affected by nutrition levels which are determined by environmental factors, including one's economic resources. As well, universalism is not synonymous with essentialism. O'Brien's work, though often categorized as such, does not constitute a return to biological essentialism once her understanding of reproduction as a biosocial process rather than brute biological event becomes clear. Such a complex understanding is key to a grasp of any materialism – including forms emerging under post-constructionism. Like for feminist standpoint epistemology debates, the question is one which emphasizes patriarchal hegemony – and is not essentialist, as Nancy Hartsock wrote: 'standpoint theory does not require feminine essentialism but rather analyses the essentialism that androcentrism attributes to women'.[16] I am struck by the ongoing relevance of O'Brien's reflection in 1984 that, 'It is odd, indeed, that we have still to argue that reproduction is a form of knowledge with

---

14   For a few see Gillian Howie, *Between Feminism and Materialism: A Question of Method*, New York: Palgrave Macmillan, 2010; Birke and Asberg, 'Biology is a feminist issue'; Kath Woodward and Sophie Woodward, *Why Feminism Matters: Feminism Lost and Found*, Basingstoke: Palgrave Macmillan, 2009; Stacy Alaimo and Susan Hekman, eds, *Material Feminisms*, Bloomington: Indiana University Press, 2008; Linda Martin Alcoff, 'Who's Afraid of Identity Politics?' in *Reclaiming Identity: Realist Theory and the Predicament of Postmodernism*, ed. Paula M.L. Moya and Michael R. Hames-Garcia. California: University of California Press, 2000, 312–44; Stevi Jackson, 'Why a Materialist Feminism is (Still) Possible – and Necessary', *Women's Studies International Forum* 24:3/4 (2001): 283–93; Noela Davis, 'New Materialism and Feminism's Anti-Biologism'; Alexandra Howson, *Embodying Gender*, London: Sage Publishers, 2005; Diana Coole and Samantha Frost, eds, *New Materialisms: Ontology, Agency, and Politics*, Durham and London: Duke University Press, 2010; Karen Barad, *Meeting the Universe Halfway: Quantum Physics and the Entanglement of Matter and Meaning*, Durham and London: Duke University Press, 2007.

15   O'Brien, *The Politics of Reproduction*, 188.

16   Hartsock, Nancy, *The Feminist Standpoint Revisited & Other Essays*, Boulder, CO: Westview Press, 1998, 233.

profound epistemological significance for women and men, and this fact is itself a massive triumph for patriarchal hegemonic practice'.[17]

Finally, revisiting O'Brien's radical reproductive materialism contributes to a growing trend in trans-disciplinary, even 'postdisciplinary' critical thought concerned with the material or ontological turn in social theory.[18] At the forefront of such thinking are Lynda Birke, Linda Alcoff, and Gillian Howie, among others. If we take feminism to be relevant even in a 'post-feminist' political climate, it is at least 'to defend rights hard won' such as legal abortion in the USA (and elsewhere), find ways to make sense of activism related to ongoing structurally entrenched, if dispersed, inequalities (for example the Slut Walks and Occupy movement), and the increasingly indisputable fact that reproductive politics are still centrally important to women (if not equally for all, and all of the time) and thus for feminist activism and theory.[19]

This book, then, is about a central paradox (of women's reproduction) as well as a central paradigm (of birth appropriation) in Western culture. Each is revealed through a recent history of feminist political theory, but both critical and more mainstream theories are rooted in Cartesian dualistic norms about women's and men's biologically determined, and mutually exclusive reproductive roles. John Stuart Mill was right that, 'ideas have consequences'. NRTs become the magnifying glass through which the paradox is writ large. In what follows I aim to provide an explanatory framework for NRTs and their paradoxically oppressive and liberating tendencies for women as potential birthers; and render intelligible birth appropriation as underpinning current Western feminist debates through dualistic understandings that are still in circulation and being negotiated in contemporary feminist praxis.

This affords the opportunity for significant theoretical advances. First, it lets us go deeper 'into and beyond' claims that postmodern arguments have been detrimental to feminism, and to carry the mantle of trans-dualism further (for example, challenging the biology/society, and sex/gender binaries).[20] Secondly, it reframes a purposive and politically engaged feminism that moves beyond blame in the academic tradition of bettering one's forebears, which can entrap its participants into a nullifying stasis.[21] This reframing includes stressing continuity and commonality while also plainly stating divergences; and finally, it allows a more generous (re)interpretation of centrally important thinkers and their contributions, and to productively reconcile them with others in the history

---

17   Mary O'Brien, 'The Commatization of Women: Patriarchal Fetishism in the Sociology of Education', *Interchange* 15:2 (1984): 57.

18   Lykke, *Feminist Studies*.

19   See Gillian Howie, *Between Feminism and Materialism*, 205; Woodward and Woodward, *Why Feminism Matters*.

20   Lykke, *Feminist Studies*, 133.

21   Zalewski, *Feminism after Postmodernism: Theorising through Practice*, London and New York: Routledge, 2000, 141.

of feminism with whom they may not otherwise be placed especially if they are positioned on opposing sides of well-established boundary lines (like the modern/postmodern one.)

My approach is hermeneutical, especially by involving *the way texts are received* as part of their overall impact. Such an interpretation 'holds that the meaning perceived in a text depends on the social setting in which it was produced as well as the social setting in which it is received and handed on'.[22] When it comes to biological determinism (but it applies to any theory), Birke claims that 'it isn't only a question of what is argued, but how that argument resonates with the wider culture' a point to give us pause when revisiting 'essentialist' theories like that of O'Brien and Hartsock, but one that is equally relevant to Judith Butler when she reflects on *Gender Trouble's* (unintended) watershed feminist anti-essentialist significance.[23]

(Re)Theorizing Reproduction

Feminist re-theorizations of reproduction must begin from Cartesian dualism that remains embedded in scholarly disciplines, especially those most influenced by postmodernism since the 1990s. In feminist theory, since the existentialist feminist Simone de Beauvoir ostensibly freed women from biologically-grounded claims of feminine inferiority by proclaiming in *The Second Sex* that 'one is not born, but rather becomes a woman', Western feminists have grappled with the challenge of reconciling female embodiment with women's autonomy and equality.[24] Bodies and their significance for women's emancipation are considered a closed chapter mainly because of widespread and effective contraceptive technologies which enables many to choose when to become pregnant. Nonetheless, for feminists in the global South, race minority women in the developed world and women with disabilities everywhere the predominating issue is the freedom to have babies.[25]

---

22   A. Clifford, 'Feminist Hermeneutics', *New Catholic Encyclopedia*, 2003. Online.

23   Birke and Asberg, 'Biology is a Feminist Issue', 417; 'Gender as Performance', in *A Critical Sense: Interviews with Intellectuals*, ed. P. Osborne, London; New York: Routledge, 1996, 111. Also as a variation on this theme, See Hemmings' *Why Stories Matter* which provides a deep analysis of the kinds of stories feminists tell themselves about where we've come from and where we're going. Two are the 'loss' and 'return' narratives which both present a problematic present feminism combined with a better past feminism that we can only hope to approximate or return to as the case may be. My intention is to avoid/subvert such simplistic and ultimately negative depictions, but I also aim partly to tell a different story while acknowledging the power of the deeply repetitive/reiterative stories we have been and continue to tell.

24   Simone De Beauvoir, *The Second Sex*, trans. H.M. Parshley, New York: Vintage Books, 1989, 267. First published in France in 1949, and in the USA in 1953.

25   Navsharan Singh, 'Contesting Reproduction; Gender, the State and Reproductive Technologies in India'. PhD Diss., Carleton University, Ottawa, 1998; Michelle Fine and

De Beauvoir's groundbreaking description of women's association with feminine essence and the corporeal as opposed to intellectual components of lived experience can be read as anti-essentialist, anti-corporeal, and anti-natal – elements bequeathed to postmodern theory, including feminist versions of postmodernism.[26] This influence was taken to its logical conclusion in Shulamith Firestone's call for the liberation of women from the 'tyranny' of biological reproduction with NRTs as developed in *The Dialectic of Sex* (1970), which I explore in Chapter 2.

This focus on gender, defined as a social construct autonomous from sex, invariably results in accusations of essentialism or false universalism whenever reproduction is raised; hence recognizing the commonalities women share because of their reproductive functions, especially in power based on marginalized characteristics, and without diminishing women's significant differences is feminism's biggest challenge. In fact, the deep rooted contradictions between motherhood and the prizing of individualist autonomy at the heart of most majoritarian-liberal feminism makes it hard to discuss many marginalized women at all.[27] Nonetheless, for most, the ability to meaningfully distinguish 'gender' from bodily sex is an academic and theoretical one. We must be able to speak about female bodies, however conscious of the risks of resurrecting an unchangeable, universal woman. Women's embodiment is only problematic in reference to Cartesian dualism, which remains entrenched in much contemporary critical theory.

I use the problematic neologism 'postmodern' to conceptualize the present terms and axes of patriarchal dualism, which was a defining feature of modern life and remains in postmodernism. While postmodern theory and practice may have had varying success destabilizing modern Cartesian and gendered duality, it is not meaningfully post-patriarchy in part because it rests on a rejection of bodies historically associated with women. To the extent that we have been unable to escape ideological constructs that pit humans against nature and men against women, for example, we remain modern; indeed, our thinking with regard to birth appropriation remains with Plato in some ways.

Amongst postmodernism's less controversial features are those associated with temporal placement (as postmodern*ity*), such as shifts in economic processes and modes of production; that is post-industrial, post-Fordist modes of production and capitalism and the blurring of geo-political border-lines both ideological and

---

Adrienne Asch, eds, *Women with Disabilities: Essays in Psychology, Culture, and Politics*, Philadelphia: Temple University Press, 1988; A. Finger, 'Claiming all of our Bodies: Reproductive Rights and Disability', in *Test-Tube Women: What Future for Motherhood?*, ed. R. Arditti, R.D. Klein and S. Minden, London: Pandora Press, 1984, 281–97.

26   For an alternative reading see the work of Toril Moi.

27   Jean Bethke Elshtain, *Public Man, Private Woman*, Princeton, NJ: Princeton University Press, 1981, 243; Amber E. Kinser, ed., *Mothering in the Third Wave*, Bradford, Ontario: Demeter Press, 2008; Sara Ruddick, *Maternal Thinking: Toward a Politics of Peace*, Boston: Beacon Press, 1995.

terrestrial associated with *globalization*. Postmodernism, then, represents shifts in focus of politics, economy and culture specifically the beginnings of a shift in political praxis from statism to globalization.[28] Furthermore, the new material situation that is expressed by the term postmodern, defines, and is defined by, new conceptions of reproduction reflected in the development and use of NRTs.

If, with due credit to Frederic Jameson, postmodernism is the 'cultural logic of late capitalism' – NRT is its technological manifestation. 'The fundamental ideological task [of postmodernism] … must remain that of coordinating new forms of practice and social and mental habits … with the new forms of economic production' associated with globalization.[29] NRTs both constitute and are constituted by a postmodern globalized capitalism which disinvests the value of whole bodies, by rationalizing its processes, in effect 'liquidizing' them as Annette Burfoot describes.[30] New reproductive technologies take part in the postmodern (reproductive) political economy whereby disembodiment enables a supply of discrete corporeal components that are readily transferable and reconstituted according to consumer reproductive needs.

In keeping with Jameson's analysis, postmodern reproduction (NRTs) allow us to function in a postmodern, globalized socio-economic milieu wherein part-time, and temporary service sector work that can easily be relocated to less-developed locales, dominates. Piecemeal work for uncertain periods of time requires a 'flexible' attitude and lifestyle to accommodate flexible production modes. NRTs allow us to respond (through postmodern techno-culture) to an economic reality that means we are less in control of our reproductive and family lives. The 'infertility' caused by a globalized capitalism – including postponement of reproduction to establish economic security – can be 'remedied' by NRTs. However, as Jameson writes, 'the interrelationship of culture and the economy here is not a one-way street but a continuous reciprocal interaction and feedback loop'[31] just as the dialectic of production and reproduction must be addressed, as they emerge in such issues as late-age first birth mothers across the affluent

---

28 See Grace Skogstad, 'Legitimacy and/or policy effectiveness? Network Governance and GMO Regulation in the European Union', *Journal of European Public Policy* 10:3 (2003): 958 for a concise discussion of economic, political and technological dimensions of globalization and their effect of undermining state-centred political authority in contemporary Canada. She writes: 'David Held and colleagues (1999) define globalization as the transformation in the spatial organization of social relations and transactions that generates flows and networks of activity and power across continents and regions'.

29 Frederic Jameson, *Postmodernism, or The Cultural Logic of Late Capitalism*, New York: Verso, 1993, xiv/xv.

30 Annette Burfoot, 'Revisiting Mary O'Brien – Reproductive Consciousness and Liquid Maternity'. Marxisms and Feminisms on the Edge, Society for Socialist Studies: Annual Meeting. Victoria, BC. June 5–7, 2013. Paper Presentation.

31 Frederic Jameson, *Postmodernism, or The Cultural Logic of Late Capitalism*, New York: Verso, 1993, xiv/xv.

Table I.1   Modern and Postmodern Reproduction

	Modern	Postmodern
Time frame	**1910–1963**	**Post-1963**
Approaches to the 'control over life'	Universal laws of reproduction	Transformation of reproductive bodies and processes to achieve a variety of goals
Reproductive processes of focus	Menstruation, contraception, abortion, birth, and menopause	Conception and (in) fertility, pregnancy, heredity, clinical genetics, male reproduction, gamete storage and donation, stem cells
Defining reproductive technology	The Pill (c1960)	In Vitro Fertilization & The Test Tube Baby
Conceptualization of the central 'problem of sex'	Fertility (in first and third worlds)	Infertility (first world only)
The body's 'nature'	Taylored. The modernist body is dictated by a particular form of industrial production method, Taylorism, that measures and controls the body's movement but also respects its internal integrity.	Tailored. The postmodernist body is characterized by a form of production that shapes and tailors the body in a way that transgresses its 'natural' bounds. That is, nature is unbounded as evident in the promise of genetic engineering and now stem cells.

capitalist countries, and a focus on infertility and low birth rates among certain demographics within them more generally.

More precisely, I use 'postmodern' to distinguish contemporary reproductive practices associated with conceptive technology from previous modern contraceptive technologies. Like Adele Clarke in *Disciplining Reproduction*, I highlight the shifting modern/postmodern parameters regarding reproductive practice and the body – in their conceptual and historical dimensions. 'Both modern and postmodern approaches to reproduction are achieved through technoscientific reconfigurations of "nature" that intervene by going "beyond the natural body"'; the main point is that they do so very differently.[32] While both approaches alter the 'natural' processes of the body, in the dominant modern approach to reproduction, the 'natural' biological body remains intact in a way that it does not with the

---

32   Adele Clarke, *Disciplining Reproduction: Modernity, American Life Sciences, and the 'Problems of Sex'*, California: University of California Press, 1998, 11.

postmodern, or new reproductive technology, a point that feminist biologist Birke makes very well in *Feminism and the Biological Body* and as Table I.1 depicts.[33]

Even though postmodernists on the surface reject the body/mind and sex/gender dualism, I show that by theorizing the body's agency as only possible through resistance to social inscription, and the body as 'materialized' through discourse, the result is a new intellectualized body, abstracted from its materiality.[34] While postmodernist theory has enriched feminist analyses and many productive conceptual advancements have resulted from their overlapping concerns, its underlying Cartesian dualism nonetheless presents a stumbling block for an embodied (rather than a discursive) material feminist theory as a matter of emphasis. For example, for some postmodern feminists a 'woman' need not be a biological female who experiences physical sensations linked to biological sex. In Butler's account, one's sex is materialized through normative social inscription.[35] In many feminist analyses since Butler, the body is similarly seen as something to be overcome through 'acting out' or 'gender performativity' something which successfully challenges heteronorms in feminist theory, but has contributed to a disintegrating effect in feminism overall.[36] While I agree with this feminist insight about the complex interaction of biological and social powers that our bodily identity instantiates, it (somewhat ironically) has heightened rather than allayed apprehensions about the material, embodied aspects of women's experience as the sex subjugated because of longstanding historical associations with nature.

For the twenty-first-century reader familiar with such postmodern theory, which often entails a post-Marxist and post-feminist stance, the terms of O'Brien's argument (rooted in Marxist and Hegelian discourse, as well as radical feminist analysis) may detract from its actual nuance and value. While I correct for the datedness of her approach in some regards, I retain the language in fidelity to her

---

33   Adapted with some modifications from Clarke, *Disciplining Reproduction*. See Lynda Birke, *Feminism and the Biological Body*, Edinburgh: Edinburgh University Press, 1999, 155, 168.

34   See for example Birke and Asberg, 'Biology is a feminist issue', 417; Noela Davis, 'New Materialism and Feminism's Anti-Biologism', 67–80; and Woodward and Woodward, *Why Feminism Matters*.

35   Judith Butler, *Gender Trouble: Feminism and the Subversion of Identity*, New York: Routledge, 1990; Judith Butler, *Bodies That Matter: On the Discursive Limits of 'Sex'*, New York: Routledge, 1993.

36   See for example, Judith Butler, 'Gender as Performance', 110; and Woodward and Woodward, *Why Feminism Matters*. Also, this is part of a more culturally situated division which has been insightfully theorized by Clare Hemmings as more of the same feminist heterosexism whereby cultural or queer theory is pitted against more empirically oriented heterosexual theory (Hemmings, *Why Stories Matter*, 91). While I am in agreement with this analysis which encourages consideration of the way texts are received as part of their overall impact, the dynamics I explore in this book are not reducible to such a paradigm. See also, Susan Stryker, 'A Conversation with Susan Stryker', *International Feminist Journal of Politics* 5:1 (March 2003): 117–29.

work and as part of the project of discursive reclamation of challenging, even contemporarily pejorative, terms.

One helpful outcome of the postmodern deconstruction of identity is the more accurate portrayal of feminist identity as multiple and dynamic, both over time and at a time. O'Brien's work has been deemed essentialist, but her universalist tone should not be taken as the whole of her argument. Nor should it eclipse what most critical scholars in other terms would readily accede to: that at the level of embodiment, itself a process (as Butler and others would agree), reproduction has been normatively inscribed hence experienced as fundamentally binary along the lines of the largely imaginary, but nonetheless embodied experience of the binary norms of 'the feminine' and 'the masculine'.

Disappearing Acts

Birth appropriation is manifest, using O'Brien's terms, in a dominating 'masculine reproductive consciousness' that disguises and seeks to control female reproductive power by positing greater masculine power. Women's embodied power is assimilated into patriarchal symbol systems and culture through attribution of women's reproductive roles to men. But reproductive consciousness is a complex biosocial concept often misunderstood, and best situated in her broader working out of feminist dialectical materialism as a fundamental feminist standpoint epistemology, although she did not use that term.

It is the notion of biosocial reproduction as a process, not a 'thing' – a dialectical reproductive materialism as captured in *her notion of reproductive consciousnesses* that is most important. O'Brien believes that men share a reproductive consciousness shaped by alienation from pregnancy and birth, and women share a disjunction between sexuality and reproduction (at least in the developed world) because of contraceptive technologies. Before reliable DNA testing only if a woman was a prisoner could men be sure their children were theirs. Contrary to most feminist theorists except O'Brien, I argue that the body/ mind and woman/man value dualism, the foundation for much patriarchal practice, is rooted in men's shared reproductive experiences and not in modern science. This goes against postmodern anti-essentialist belief but is a crucial starting point for understanding reproduction and politics, and associated contemporary feminist debates.

NRTs are a new instantiation of an old paradigm of birth appropriation because they conceptually and physically disembody reproductive process by removing significant aspects of reproduction from the female body, fundamentally changing our understanding of humans' relationship to nature. For women, moreover, although contraceptive technologies separate sex and reproduction, NRTs enable separation of reproduction and parenthood. Both represent experiences from the perspective of men's reproductive consciousnesses. Drawing on O'Brien's theory of dialectical reproductive materialism, I explore the consequences of the material change NRTs produce in the birthing process, and their effects on the social relations of reproduction and women's reproductive consciousnesses. It is also important to understand the material, social, and ideational practices out of which NRTs were developed and which continue to support such technologies through disembodiment of women. Postmodernism, especially because it represents an intertwined anti-epistemological and anti-methodological dimension in feminism is part of the structure of power/knowledge relations which supports and enables NRTs, further alienating women from their bodies in a misguided attempt to avoid the consequences of reproduction.[37]

It is equally significant that women have readily incorporated NRTs into their lives and that feminist theory has had to incorporate changing understandings of the 'nature' of the body (and Cartesian dualism). Indeed, as many feminists (including O'Brien) have argued, the shifts in material process that reproductive technologies inaugurate are not clearly negative for women. Just as we have all consumed, literally and for our immediate gain, food technologies that perpetuate global inequalities. The consequences of technologies vary, depending on socio-cultural and political factors. Technology always has unintended consequences. So although NRTs help women better 'control' their own reproduction, they simultaneously enable others to do so, too, especially because NRTs disembody reproductive processes and further mechanize reproduction. They are not wholly determined by the context from whence they come, nor neutral tools; they are designed as solutions to certain problems so originate from and serve particular values and perceptions. For example, what gets selected as the problems NRTs are seen to provide the answers to reflects specific historical and political values, and moreover, specific articulations of these; therefore women's bodies belong in a patriarchal history as well as in a feminist theoretical lineage that influences, and is also influenced by, the former. Questions about women's bodily differences from men (and other women), and their cultural and political significance are at the centre of feminist thought and activism. Different conceptualizations of the nature of the body, especially whether it is socially constructed or natural, have altered with cultural milieu and suggested distinct feminist strategies, just as social theory relating to the nature/nurture debate in feminism was dominated since the nineties by a postmodern view but is beginning to change in the material turn inaugurated by the emergence of postconstructionist, material feminisms.

My goal in this book is to bring the body and sex back into serious feminist analysis. I believe feminism can represent women's manifold corporeal experiences, especially of those who do not conform to the Anglo-Saxon, heterosexual, able-bodied, and economically privileged norm, yet find the unity in this diversity. O'Brien's understanding of reproductive experience as biosocial is useful here as are a number of materialist feminists who build from the same onto-epistemological base like Birke, Alcoff, and disability theorist Rosemarie Garland-Thomson. The moments of reproductive experience she theorizes are

---

37   Lykke, *Feminist Studies*.

dialectical, not merely biological facts, but also socio-culturally mediated. We have an element of control over them: women know what they are doing when giving birth, even if it is involuntary. In the same way, the body is material, i.e. it is biological, even as it is mediated socially and culturally.

Sex is not an either/or, *either* socially constructed *or* a biologically determined event. In other words, there is a complex interchange of the biological and historical in reproduction as O'Brien, Hartsock and other materialist feminists have argued. Insofar as reproduction is (at least partly) biological, it is part of the 'material' realm – biological nature comprehended in human thought and practice' which is dialectically structured.[38] It is the sociocultural inscription of sexed bodies that lends a normative determinism to the biological. Yet ironically as Butler reveals, this is also an opportunity for normative subversion.[39]

I do not wish to re-evaluate gender binary as radical feminists did, or proliferate sex/gender identities as postmoderns have done. This attempt is signified in the reconceptualization of the terms sex and gender as *sex/gender* to represent the inextricably intertwined character of the biological and the cultural if we may, at least hypothetically, speak of them as distinct and autonomous concepts.[40] This interaction between sex and gender represents a deeper way of understanding both commonality and difference, and represents an attempt to mitigate nature/nurture polarization and its effects by focusing on the biosocial approach to embodiment and identity.

Ultimately, the book demonstrates that feminist (like mainstream) political theorists in the West have abandoned 'the body' in its material dimensions and in doing so, contribute to patriarchal hegemony based on Cartesian dualism. I call for a re-membering of the material dimensions of bodies and their political and philosophical significance by mediating various instantiations of such dualism that is so deeply entrenched in Western culture and politics that they become almost invisible. This includes a recognition of the bodies of those that most challenge oppressive cultural norms by representing all that we would deny; that is, our mortal origins and lack of 'control', disease, death and suffering/disability. These experiences, including pregnancy and birth, I argue highlight dependency and interdependency, which despite their negative connotation in Western societies, are not accurately understood as opposite to independence and autonomy (hence

---

38   Mary O'Brien, *Reproducing the World: Essays in Feminist Theory*, Boulder, CO: Westview Press, 1989, 236–7.

39   Butler, *Gender Trouble*; Butler, *Bodies That Matter*.

40   Gayle Rubin, 'The Traffic in Women: Notes on the "Political Economy" of Sex', in *Toward an Anthropology of Women*, ed. Rayna Reiter, New York: Monthly Review Press, 1975; Jill Vickers, 'Whatever Happened to Sex?', *Canadian Woman Studies* 18:4 (Winter 1999): 115; Mary O'Brien, *The Politics of Reproduction*. See also Lykke, *Feminist Studies* for her similar conceptualization of 'gender/sex'.

to be avoided) but fundamental to the profoundly humanizing (if undeniably paradoxical) potential of material corporeality.[41]

Overview

The paradox of women's reproduction in the age of new reproductive technologies is that with increasing material disembodiment of reproductive processes, men's and women's physiological differences are potentially mitigated, which can have progressive effects, but only where patriarchal practice is similarly altered. Although these changes may 'free' women from embodied reproduction (and its associated roles) they also further naturalize men's embodied reproductive experiences of the separation between sex and reproduction, and pregnancy and parenthood; in essence, of bio/physiological act and social role. With NRTS and DNA testing, for example, men's and women's differences in reproduction are radically altered; men can technologically mediate their paternal uncertainty, and women's reproductive processes (and maternal certainty) can be disembodied by NRTs. Androcentric dualism is not automatically challenged in the development and use of NRTs and has a significant reinforcing role in a continuous history of birth appropriation.

In Part I, Reproduction in the Twenty-first Century, I explain, develop and substantiate my claim that NRTs represent an unprecedented reproductive disembodiment with profound implications. This significant moment of reproductive change is a paradoxical offering for women but is ultimately to be approached with caution because it is part of an ongoing dualistic conceptual framework built upon women's and men's differing reproductive physiology and its normative patriarchal qualifications. In Chapter 1 I frame new reproductive technology as a way of seeing the world that contributes to a new conceptual, collective, and individual experience of disembodiment, especially for women. I develop the claim that this disembodiment is fundamentally androcentric since based on men's inability to conceive, gestate and give birth. To clarify the practical, legal and social significance of such disembodiment I highlight its visual and discursive manifestations and focus on its political implications.

In Part II, Feminism and New Reproductive Technologies, I argue that women's reproductive consciousnesses are shaped on a number of levels, by a history of birth appropriation based on patriarchal dualism. Feminists have theorized and resisted different politically entrenched sex/gender regimes, developing ideologies and strategies with regard to the relationships between nature and convention; but can feminists subvert patriarchal dualism at the heart of varying sex/gender regimes upheld by states? Feminists approach the disembodiment of women's

---

41   See especially Whitney's 'Dependency Relations'. This is a belief with a long tradition in feminist ethics of care and feminist critiques of liberal individualism, and feminist theories of relational autonomy more generally.

reproductive processes wrought by NRTs in at least three distinct, if interrelated, ways: resistance to, embrace of, and equivocal regarding the technologies. In chapters 2 and 3, I evaluate each position on the basis of its ability to transcend patriarchal dualism in its often underlying treatment of the man/technology over woman/nature value binary in modern Western societies which is associated with distinct views about the unmediated body's status as burdensome or freeing.

Chapter 2 explores two seemingly oppositional forms of feminist discourse that have emerged in response to NRTs since the 1980s. Feminists who embrace the technology and are rooted in the radical materialist feminist manifesto of Firestone respond quite differently from the feminists who resist NRTs and are inspired by the radical and eco-feminist principles of such thinkers as Germaine Greer and Vandana Shiva. Feminist resistors who were most active during roughly 1984–1991 constitute a 'first phase' of feminist critique of NRTs. The key distinction is between this first phase which is largely, though not wholly, defined by explicit resistance to NRTs and a 'second phase' (roughly 1992–2001) coinciding with the linguistic turn in social science of the late 1980s/early 1990s and influenced by it. Both responses are found to ultimately reinforce problematic dualism by, in principle, either embracing technology to overcome the limits of the 'natural' body, or resisting the technology on the basis of the maintenance of a 'natural' or otherwise essentialized body.

In Chapter 3, equivocal feminists constitute a third categorical response to NRTs which incorporates elements of both the embracing and resisting feminist responses while critiquing the oppositional and dualistic frameworks presented in each. While they tend to adopt a social constructionist view of 'the body', (as in our biological roots) like Hobbes, they perceive it as neither naturally oppressive, nor necessarily liberating. I demonstrate how their arguments and critiques of the previous positions amount to a mediation of the social and biological arguments of the embracers and resistors, respectively. I conclude that, of the three feminist responses to NRTs, the equivocal response represents the most promising approach to bypass the problematic patriarchal dualism at the heart of disembodying NRTs because it entails a biosocial understanding of reproduction akin to that of O'Brien and the new material feminists that undermines the nature/culture duality.

Part III explores Material Resolutions to the biosocial dialectic examined throughout the book. In Chapter 4 I return to O'Brien's complex conception of biosocial reproduction as a mediation of the patriarchal nature/culture dualism, linking her insights to standpoint feminism and the new material feminisms as constituting a post-constructionist 'thinking technology' to highlight what they enable in feminist thought as a trans-dualist analytic framework.[42] I draw on recent literature which examines the new material feminisms (variously referred to) as part of an emerging multidisciplinary field of scholarship in which feminist theory is prominent, and which begins from a critique of the limits of social

---

42   Lykke, 'The Timeliness of Post-Constructionism'.

constructionism (but also of biological determinism) in favor of a more complex material analysis.

In Chapter 5 and the Conclusion I outline potential feminist resolutions to a history of patriarchal dualism manifest in birth appropriation by theorizing the 'new' material feminisms as a methodology that is trans-dualistic in the same sense of O'Brien's biosocial reproduction. Chapters 4 and 5 frame the new material feminisms as a post-constructionist 'thinking technology', and focuses on what they enable in feminist thought as 'breaking feminist waves' and more broadly, as a trans-disciplinary, trans-dualistic theoretical framework with radical epistemological and methodological potential for addressing disembodying sexist dualism. More specifically, the new material feminisms begin from the same conceptual renegotiation as well as O'Brien's biosocial reproduction and can be seen to constitute a new methodology that can mitigate the modern/postmodern, or (biological) essentialism/(social) constructionism impasse in feminist theory. I propose that post-constructionism entails a methodology capable of mitigating nature/culture duality in its overlapping but divergent domains; most significantly, in feminist theory, especially the social constructionist/biological essentialist impasse linked to debates about new reproductive technologies.

In the Conclusion I re-visit questions about the significance of NRTs in the context of women's reproduction as a central paradox, and birth appropriation as a central paradigm, in Western culture and suggest interventions in contemporary reproduction at the conceptual level that may address birth appropriation rather than further it building on the trans-dualism that emerges from feminist responses to new reproductive technologies with reference to the equivocal feminist position.

PART I
Reproduction in the Twenty-first Century

Chapter 1
New Reproductive Technologies and Disembodiment

In this chapter I shall investigate a third moment of 'world historically' significant change in reproductive process as evident in the distinctions between the mass contraceptive technology of Mary O'Brien's era and the conceptive and other new reproductive technology of mine. The latter is part of the globalization of capitalism evident in the biotechnology revolution and includes industrialized agriculture as well as the commercialization of medicine. I build upon the work of this long-time midwife turned political theorist as an interpretive framework for those conceptive technologies that enable new choices for women and profoundly alter the material and normative milieu in which they might exercise them.

In theorizing a third moment of change in reproductive praxis, I retain the designation 'world historical' significance in the senses of a change in the dialectical social, ideational, and material aspects of reproduction; and of a shift in the human to nature relationship which creates a critical distance from and new perspective on reproduction, especially for women. New reproductive technology is a 'new' moment because it alters, once again, the material experience of reproductive process by estranging the reproducer from nature because it involves disembodiment of reproductive process. Conceptive reproductive technologies (physically and conceptually) take human reproduction outside women's bodies. While contraceptive technologies let women choose *not* to bear children, at least in ideal circumstances and for some women, new reproductive technologies (NRT) take this for granted and add new choices for women; whether to have children, when and how to have those children; and increasingly what kind of children to have. NRTs are a new form of rationalization of reproductive process that is increasingly interventionist in bodily processes and alters our understandings of reproduction.

NRT, using O'Brien's concept, involves a further 'transformation in human consciousness of human relations with the natural world'.[1] Arguably since the discovery of paternity, but certainly since Aristotle, men have understood themselves to be apart from and above nature, whereas women have been considered close to nature.[2] But with NRTs, women have begun to alienate

---

1   Mary O'Brien, *The Politics of Reproduction*, Boston: Routledge and Kegan Paul, 1981, 22.

2   Carolyn Merchant, *The Death of Nature: Women, Ecology and the Scientific Revolution*, San Francisco: Harper San Francisco, 1980; Carolyn Merchant, 'Ecofeminism

themselves from nature, and to relate to it more like men, who often understand themselves as distinct from, if not in opposition to, it. This realignment radically alters women's material experiences of reproductive process and consciousnesses such that women may be 'liberated' by it; at the same time, they may become more deeply estranged and alienated from reproduction. Consider, for example, the recent consideration in Ontario, Canada to make a C-section an elective procedure as opposed to a strictly medically necessary one.[3] Such practices are emblematic of the experience of reproduction as increasingly technological; the central metaphor for women's reproductive bodies in such a time is one of 'separation' leading Arditti to conclude, 'We are now at the point where biological motherhood is in question and in need of explicit definition, just like fatherhood used to be'.[4]

Significantly, with conceptive technology women can both separate sex from reproduction and reproduce without intercourse, which has long been possible for men as sperm donors.[5] For example, women can donate their eggs in the same way, giving rise to legal situations that disadvantage and devalue the pregnant 'surrogate' mother's contribution, denying her parental rights, which accrue to the 'real' parents who are the gamete donors. Equally problematic, a recent New Jersey ruling collapsed distinctions between traditional (genetic) and gestational surrogacy, adopting what some would call paternalistic moral tones that pre-empt women's choices, including to act as surrogate mothers.[6]

Conceptive technology provides the conditions for a heightened displacement of reproduction from women, who in unmediated procreation have a dominant role, to other interests including states, the medical industrial complex, and techno-science. As O'Brien understood, the commodification of women is a central feature of this displacement. Ingrid Makus explains that this is why many feminists endorse old reproductive technologies (especially abortion) but oppose NRTs. The contradiction presented by NRTs for feminists is that they simultaneously reinforce the separation between sex and reproduction which many feminists believe provides women greater control over their bodies, yet are a part of another moment that threatens their reproductive autonomy. '[T]he new

---

and Feminist Theory', in *Environmental Ethics*, ed. Michael Boylan, Upper Saddle River, NJ: Prentice Hall, 2001, 76–83; and Carolyn Merchant, 'Mining the Earth's Womb', in *Philosophy of Technology: The Technological Condition: An Anthology*, ed. Robert C. Scharff and Val Dusek, Malden, MA: Blackwell Publishers, 2003, 417–28.

3   Abby Lippman, 'C-section fight does a U-turn', *Globe and Mail*, 3 March 2004, A21.

4   Rita Arditti, 'Commercializing Motherhood', in *The Politics of Motherhood: Activist Voices from Left to Right*, ed. Alexis Jetter, Annelise Orleck and Diana Taylor, Hanover, NH: University Press of New England, 1997, 322–33.

5   Arditti, 'Commercializing Motherhood', 322.

6   Stephanie Saul, 'New Jersey Judge Calls Surrogate Legal Mother of Twins', *The New York Times*, 31 December 2009; Alex Blaze, 'New Jersey Court Decides against Gestational Surrogacy Contracts', *The Bilerico Project*, 5 January 2010.

reproductive technologies, by introducing new players into the game ... threaten to diffuse women's first access to the "new life", dispersing it among physicians and medical researchers'.[7]

Furthermore, the disembodiment of NRTs and commodification of women's bodies heighten present inequalities between women, such as economically disadvantaged minority women who provide various services to usually Caucasian middle class women, who can afford them. A clear global example of this ethically fraught scenario is evident in 'reproductive tourism', which offers prospective parents the ability to pay for reproductive services in countries where the economic costs are lower than their home country. For example, in Mumbai, India, prospective parents from Britain or the US can find a surrogate mother for about a third of the cost at home. On the other hand, the surrogate's fee of about $7,500 is more than they would otherwise make in fifteen years.[8]

The social relations of reproduction that can mediate the newest forms of alienation engendered in NRTs have not yet emerged, although one response is clear in many women's and feminists' flight from the body. The new social relations of reproduction and the female and male reproductive consciousnesses to accompany the material experiences of the new reproductive technology will reflect its paradoxical nature: conceptive technology offers a greater degree of technological control over the processes of reproduction which can be perceived as a threat to the embodied integrity of women who bear children, and also as potential liberation of women from the toils of traditionally conceived heteronormative sexuality and reproduction including traditional reproductive ages. The use of NRT will, undoubtedly, liberate some women who would otherwise be unable to reproduce biologically. I wish, however, to problematize the material transformation of reproductive praxis within a socio-historical context of patriarchal hegemony, especially regarding the domination of a problematic androcentric liberal 'equality' discourse and legal framework.

Technology as Theory (or 'a way of seeing')

Technology fundamentally affects how we understand our world and our place within it. As Jacques Ellul says, 'when technique enters into every area of life ... it ceases to be external to man and becomes his very substance. It is no longer face to face with man but is integrated with him, and it progressively absorbs him'.[9]

---

7 Ingrid Makus, *Women, Politics and Reproduction: The Liberal Legacy*, Toronto: University of Toronto Press, 1996, 142.

8 Michael Sandel, Transcripts for 'Lecture 2: Morality in Politics', *BBC Reith Lectures: A New Citizenship*, 16 June 2009. http://www.bbc.co.uk/programmes/b00kt7rg.

9 Cited in Heather Menzies, *Canada in the Global Village*, Ottawa: Carleton University Press, 1997, 37.

Most importantly, what we consider 'natural' changes.[10] We become less capable of critical reflection because the technologies become a fundamental part of our lives and consciousness. When Marshall McLuhan stated that 'the medium is the message'[11] he captured how the significance of technological change was not in a particular technology's 'apparent content' for example '(the transportation that a car provides or the news program that the television supplies) but in the systemic changes that they catalyze'.[12] Consequently, the more meaningful questions raised by technology have to do with the constitution of the self and his or her environment: 'How does it alter our experience of everyday life? How does it change our concepts of self, community, politics, nature, time, distance?'[13]

NRTs refer to any of the 'conditions, technologies, procedures and practices' that contribute to the creation, gestation, and birthing of (human) life outside the female body.[14] 'New' reproductive technologies are distinguished from 'old' reproductive technologies in terms of their focus on the (technologically-mediated) creation of new life (conception, gestation, and birth) rather than intervention in its (embodied) creation through contraception and abortion. At times I use 'conceptive technology' interchangeably with NRTs since biotech's relocation of conception is what is new about NRTs, though they are referred to differently in various legal or policy contexts, for example, 'assisted reproductive technologies', (in Canada) and 'human assisted reproductive technologies' (in New Zealand).

There are many grey areas when comparing disparate technologies under the banner of 'disembodiment' which can be clarified by understanding the many dimensions of disembodiment. The technologies I include under the rubric 'NRTs' vary widely in terms of their level of technological intervention and routine use. For instance, the process of egg extraction for IVF is quite different from ultrasound imaging. However, it is clear that ultrasound (especially the newer 3 and 4D varieties) is part of conceptual disembodiment because it enables a foetocentric worldview that is separate from the pregnant woman's and has coincided with a rise in perception of a foetus/embryo as a rights-bearing individual, something that Valerie Hartouni has termed 'the visual discourse of foetal autonomy'.[15]

---

10   Valerie Hartouni, *Cultural Conceptions: On Reproductive Technologies and the Remaking of Life*, Minneapolis: University of Minnesota Press, 1997.

11   Marshall McLuhan, *Understanding Media: The Extensions of Man*, London: Routledge, 1967.

12   Jerry Mander, 'Technologies of Globalization', in *The Case Against the Global Economy And For a Turn Toward the Local*, ed. Jerry Mander and Edward Goldsmith, San Francisco: Sierra Club Books, 1996, 345.

13   Mander, 'Technologies of Globalization', 345.

14   Government Services Canada, *Proceed With Care: Final Report of the Royal Commission on New Reproductive Technologies*, Ottawa, Canada: Minister of Government Services Canada, 1993, 4.

15   Hartouni, *Cultural Conceptions*, 67. See also an excellent discussion of the conflation of 'seeing and knowing' associated with 3 and 4 dimensional sonograms in Julie

While there are good reasons to evaluate reproductive technologies separately I address them thematically. I recognize that different reproductive technologies involve 'separate emotional and physical dilemmas', have different 'social meaning', and even within a particular category (i.e. contraceptive or conceptive technology) vary widely in terms of the level of intervention in the body (for example diaphragm versus tubal litigation); I also see the need for comprehensive frameworks for assessment, especially regarding NRTs and birth appropriation.[16]

(Dis) embodiment

The term 'embodiment' conveys the boundaries of human corporeality that are the condition of possibility for one's relative autonomy and community. I draw from Lisa Mitchell's useful discussion of 'embodied perception' where she distinguishes between the 'body ... defined as "a biological, material entity"', and 'embodiment as "the existential condition of possibility for culture and self"'.[17] Embodiment also signifies the interplay of biological and social forces in construction of gendered selfhood, identity, and agency. To be an embodied self, or subject, acknowledges the rootedness of subjective experience in bodies that are lived out materially, but never wholly determined by their biological features. This suggests that embodiment involves a perceived/perceiving self-inseparable from its body in any complete sense (out of body experiences and plastic surgery aside), and the possibility of making autonomous decisions about what happens to that body, as far as is possible.

While the body implies at least partial autonomy of a self-legislating and self-governing being, embodiment means that each is discursively linked to others (collectively and individually). Subjectivity arises in awareness of this separation and connectedness, but it also defies Cartesian dualism for there is no true separation between one's body and one's self. Mitchell notes that 'A central assumption of this approach is that "our bodies are not objects to us ... [rather] they are an integral part of the perceiving subject"'.[18] This perception affects self and other in an inter-constitutive fashion. While an element of control over the way one's body is perceived (and one perceives others') may be a fundamental and desirable component of embodiment, as social creatures we cannot escape various historically contingent and normative interpretations of our material features.

Palmer's 'Seeing and Knowing: Ultrasound Images in the Contemporary Abortion Debate', *Feminist Theory* 10 (2009): 173–89.

16   Nancy Lublin, *Pandora's Box: Feminism Confronts Reproductive Technology*, Lanham, MD: Rowman and Littlefield Publishers, Inc., 1998, 2–3.

17   Lisa M. Mitchell, *Baby's First Picture: Ultrasound and the Politics of Fetal Subjects*, Toronto: University of Toronto Press, 2001, 15.

18   Mitchell, *Baby's First Picture*, 15.

Furthermore, others' bodies are an integral part of our own, not only materially (as hereditary genetics, and pregnancy makes clear at one extreme) but also psycho-discursively/psycho-socially (as, for example, with inherited lifestyle, beliefs, and culture). Sara Ahmed aptly challenges 'the body' as a concept of the singular, privatized/individualized self. Drawing on Gail Weiss's claim that 'to be embodied is to be capable of being affected by other bodies'[19] or, in a word, *inter-embodiment,* she builds on the claim that 'the lived experience of embodiment is always already *the social experience of dwelling with other bodies*'.[20] Our embodied experiences, she argues, are fundamentally social as a necessary condition for experiencing ourselves as separate and unique, something many feminist theorists and other contemporary philosophers such as Charles Taylor have explored.[21] Women's reproductive potentialities put them in a counter-hegemonic subject position, both as actual and as potential birth-givers in patriarchal cultures built on gender binaries. Women, as those who hold the potential to be other than individual (literally, 'one who cannot be divided') are *de facto* epistemological outsiders in Western cultures rooted in liberal political thought.

One branch of Western feminism has long argued for the inter-constitutive relationship of bodies and selves. It is significant that the most internationally successful Western feminist export was the Boston Health Collective's *Our Bodies Ourselves* (1969) which, as the title implies, promotes a view that for women the body is an 'intrinsic part of the self'.[22] Announcing the women's health movement in second wave feminism, it came with the politicized message that having control over your body was synonymous with being in control of yourself. Wendi Hadd rejects the discourse of women's 'control', adopted by feminists in reproductive debates because it perpetuates a mind/body dualism that is inimical to their aims. She writes, 'The body is not only a physical manifestation of the self but an integral component of the self, it is not just where we live but an element of our living'.[23] In truth, then, we cannot 'control' ourselves since 'we' are not separate from our physical selves; and we ought to prioritize this integrated experience of

19   Sara Ahmed, *Strange Encounters: Embodied Others in Post-Coloniality*, New York: Routledge, 2000, 47.

20   Ahmed, *Strange Encounters*, 47.

21   This is a part of a history of the self in feminist theory: 'the relational self' which includes relations with others using such terms as 'inter-relationality', and 'relational theories of autonomy' (Witt, *The Metaphysics of Gender*, 201). Furthermore, these concepts are at the heart of feminist ethics of care, feminist standpoint epistemology especially as a communitarian critique of individual autonomy as an erroneous starting point in liberal theory. See also Charles Taylor, *The Ethics of Authenticity*, Cambridge, MA: Harvard University Press, 1991; Charles Taylor, *Multiculturalism and the 'Politics of Recognition'*, Princeton, NJ: Princeton University Press, 1992.

22   Kath Woodward and Sophie Woodward, *Why Feminism Matters: Feminism Lost and Found*, Basingstoke: Palgrave Macmillan, 2009, 63.

23   Wendi Hadd, 'A Womb with a View: Women as Mothers and the Discourse of the Body', *Berkeley Journal of Sociology* 36 (1991): 165–75, 173.

corporeality as a matter of principle. This argument, properly understood, performs a trans-dualistic understanding of the body that combines Mitchell's concepts of body and embodiment. Furthermore, its most important implications stem from insisting on the agency of the biological body which is similar to O'Brien's biosocial understanding of reproduction, and is also evident in recent articulations of embodiment in the new material feminisms.

At the heart of many feminist critiques of NRTs, is that they disembody women and can thus de-subjectify them on at least two levels; by taking female reproductive process outside of women (for example by physically taking conception out with IVF and ET) and presenting the embryo as a 'free-floating' entity (with ultrasound and imaging technologies). Both are linked to the displacement of women's epistemological standpoint as potential birth-givers. The subject position associated with women's embodied reproduction as one of interconnection with another developing corporeality, is delegitimized and displaced with other logics – specifically that of the individual at the foundation of liberal narratives of personhood.

The sociopolitical and cultural context of NRTs is characterized by a focus on the scientific and male contribution to conception, gestation, and birth, which facilitates the perception of the embryo/foetus as a separate-from-the-mother 'rights' bearing subject whose legally defended needs may be in conflict with the woman in whose body it resides. This technologically-assisted, foetocentric, and androcentric reading of reproduction constitutes a de-centring and devaluation of women's reproductive role and threatens their subjectivity and autonomy while pregnant. As a corrective measure, Imogen Tyler asserts: 'the production of a visual vocabulary of pregnant subjectivity is necessary to challenge "the visual discourse of foetal autonomy"'.[24]

Visual

The way that NRT 'disembodies' and its detrimental consequences for the statuses of women are best seen with ultrasound technology, which is a direct link from the outside world connecting doctor to baby, in effect erasing the woman's body. A number of issues raised by disembodiment are revealed in ultrasound technology. Furthermore, the cultural/political dimensions of creating a reception for NRTs may also be seen.

Many theorists have noted that as the foetus becomes more clearly visualized through NRTs, the female body as an organic whole required for its existence is rendered invisible.[25] This often takes the form of conceptually representing the

---

24 Imogen Tyler, 'Reframing Pregnant Embodiment', in *Transformations: Thinking Through Feminism*, ed. Sara Ahmed, Janet Kilby, Celia Lury, Maureen McNeil and Beverley Skeggs, London and New York: Routledge, 2000, 300.

25 For example, Susan Merrill Squier, 'Fetal Subjects and Maternal Objects: Reproductive Technology and the New Fetal/Maternal Relation', *The Journal of Medicine*

female body as parts required for reproduction.[26] Visualizing the embryo/foetus inside the pregnant woman's body shifts the focus from her, without whom the embryo/foetus could not exist, to the embryo/foetus as its own separate entity. Ultrasound enables an enhanced subjectivization of the foetus and an associated ambiguity surrounding the maternal subject as Susan Squier writes: 'Objectified, constituted as antagonist to a pre-eminent gene/embryo/foetus, the maternal subject is disturbingly difficult to ascertain, articulate or affirm'.[27] As a necessary counterpoint, however, Julie Palmer argues that such technology, especially in its newer 3 and 4D development, by presenting a very clear image of the placenta and umbilical cord holds the potential for lay viewers to 'think[ing] differently about the interconnections – material and social – between pregnant women and foetuses and to relocate women as the subjects of their pregnancies'.[28]

Ultrasound (and other monitoring/visualizing) technology not only made possible the rise in public perception of the foetus as separate from the mother's body, but also a displacement of women-centred understandings of pregnancy by 'the public pregnancy'.[29] For example, Squier writes, 'Whereas once the interior space of the woman was unavailable to the scientific gaze, and pregnancy was marked by the woman's testimony that she had felt the foetus move, now the woman's own internal foetal movement is relegated to the unvoiced and unwarranted realm of private experience, while the interior space of the woman

---

and Philosophy 21:5 (1996): 515–35; Susan Merrill Squier, *Babies in Bottles: Twentieth-Century Visions of Reproductive Technology*, New Brunswick, New Jersey: Rutgers University Press, 1994; Susan Merrill Squier, *Liminal Lives: Imagining the Human at the Frontiers of Biomedicine*, Durham, NC: Duke University Press, 2004; Rosalind Pollack Petchesky, 'Foetal Images: The Power of Visual Culture in the Politics of Reproduction', in *Reproductive Technologies: Gender, Motherhood and Medicine*, ed. Michelle Stanworth, Minneapolis: University of Minnesota Press, 1987, 57–80; Mitchell, *Baby's First Picture*; Sarah Franklin, 'Postmodern Procreation: A Cultural Account of Assisted Reproduction', in *Conceiving the New World Order: The Global Politics of Reproduction*, ed. Faye D. Ginsburg and Rayna Rapp, Berkeley: University of California Press, 1995, 323–45; Sarah Franklin, *Embodied Progress: A Cultural Account of Assisted Conception*, London: Routledge, 1997; Carol A. Stabile, *Feminism and the Technological Fix*, Manchester: Manchester University Press, 1994; Karen Barad, 'Getting Real: Technoscientific Practices and the Materialization of Reality', *Differences: A Journal of Feminist Cultural Studies* 10:2 (1998): 87–128, cited in *Material Feminisms*, ed. Stacy Alaimo and Susan Hekman, Bloomington: Indiana University Press, 2008, 18.

26   For example, Mitchell, William Arney and Ann Oakley argue that 'ultrasound transforms pregnant women from embodied, thinking, and knowledgeable individuals into 'maternal environments', or tissue that may or may not yield a clear ultrasound image' (Mitchell, *Baby's First Picture*, 20).

27   Squier, 'Fetal Subjects and Maternal Objects', 532.

28   Julie Palmer, 'The Placental Body in 4D: Everyday Practices of Non-Diagnostic Sonography', *Feminist Review* 93 (2009): 64–80.

29   Anne Balsamo cited in Squier, 'Fetal Subjects and Material Objects', 519.

is available for all to see as part of the technologized state'[30] Similarly, Mitchell demonstrates that ultrasound has become a routine part of pre-natal medical care that does not require the 'patient's' consent.[31] While the emphasis on seeing, rather than women's embodied sensations, in reproductive techno-science is critiqued by many, it is not by all. Petchesky for example, writes that, 'to suggest that feeling is somehow more natural than seeing contradicts women's changing historical experience'. Nonetheless I am persuaded by the view that the normative ubiquity of such technology tends toward women's self-alienation from embodied corporeality during reproduction.[32]

Furthermore, this technology continues to develop, has been commercialized and builds on politically entrenched anti-choice narratives. In the US ultrasound technology is at the centre of a 'prenatal portrait business'.[33] In Canada's national news magazine, *Macleans*, the writers proclaim under the caption 'Dancing Baby' that 3D ultrasound reveals that 'at twelve weeks babies yawn and walk. At 26 they scratch, cry and hiccup'.[34] This humanization of the embryo/foetus defies the principles of basic embryology, not to mention common sense. Most recently in the US with so-called 'The Women's Right to Know' legislation in Texas and Louisiana – women seeking an abortion will undergo mandatory ultrasound imaging, followed by a waiting period. Additionally, Julie Palmer has written of how the 3D sonogram has been 'widely reported as new evidence for a reduction in the gestational time limit'.[35] Significantly, she argues that the clarity of the image to the untrained eye contributes to a conflation of 'seeing and knowing' in the public discourse of citizen rights, which arms lay people with a false sense of medico-scientific competence to buttress their moral principles.

Images of foetuses *in utero* and the embryonic pose have long been part of our cultural landscape, creating an environment ripe for foeto-centric politics and technologies. Popular culture exploits the image of the embryo enabled by ultrasound to sell everything from electronics (Future Shop) and music (compact disc covers) to cosmetics (skin care products) and real estate (the *Ottawa Express* newspaper). These images, it could be argued, are harmless because the maternal/foetal relationship is assumed; however, in a time when 'pro-life' abortion politics can be deadly and women's rights to abortion remain unstable, retractable, or

---

30　Squier, 'Fetal Subjects and Maternal Objects', 519. See also Barbara Duden who argues in her study of eighteenth-century Germany that before visualization technologies, pregnancy was a (fittingly) woman-centred affair (Cited in Squier, 'Fetal Subjects and Maternal Objects', 518.)

31　Mitchell, *Baby's First Picture*.

32　See Hadd, 'A Womb With A View', 172.

33　Rita Kempley, 'Prenatal Pictures: Womb for Trouble? A growing trend has some worried about this use of ultrasound', *The Washington Post*, 18 August 2003, 1.

34　'Dancing Baby', *Macleans*, 12 July 2004, 12.

35　Julie Palmer, 'Seeing and Knowing: Ultrasound images in the contemporary abortion debate', *Feminist Theory* 10:2 (2009): 173–84.

absent, any representation of an embryo or foetus as an autonomous being has political consequences. Anti-abortion activists have used ultrasound pictures on picket signs and as central to their campaigns to argue for the right-to-life of foetuses and embryos. Hartouni clarifies the role of the image of the free-floating foetus in the 1980s when 'legislative efforts [were made] to redefine constitutional language, broaden the meaning of the word person, and give concrete reality to the idea of "fetus as person"',[36] She links anti-abortion legislative efforts with popular visual discourse in the form of ubiquitous foetal images in the public arena usually accompanied by written text that 'might pose a question ('Aren't they forgetting someone?'), make an assertion ('Unborn babies are people too'), or issue a call to action ('Stop the killing!')'.[37]

Discursive

Women are also disembodied as they become increasingly absent from medical and popular discourse and images of birth/reproduction, or are spoken of as body parts, rather than the central subjects of pregnancy. Michelle Stanworth, by drawing attention to who is the subject and who the object in NRT literature, argues that women's reproductive agency is being dismantled by being decentred. 'The focus of the new conceptive technologies is not really "infertility" ... nor is it even "the family". Ultimately, the focus is "babies" and their precursors, foetuses'.[38]

Stanworth reveals how the very terms used regarding NRTs, as implicitly androcentric and feto-centric, eclipse a pregnant woman's part in childbearing. For example, the phrase '"test-tube baby" conjures an odd image of a foetus growing independently of the body of a woman', which is simply inaccurate (but not innocent).[39] Similarly, insemination is only 'artificial' in how the semen makes contact with the ovum, '[b]ut a natural process of conception still occurs, if it occurs, within the woman's body'.[40] Like many other feminist theorists, Stanworth also deconstructs how surrogacy degrades a pregnant woman's role in creating the new life: '[a] woman who goes through a pregnancy, and gives birth to an infant, can only be a "surrogate" if pregnancy itself does not count as an act of mothering'.[41] As I argue, Stanworth implies that scientific, medical, and social scientific discourse that focuses on the embryo/foetus as separate from the pregnant woman, and describes birth in a way that involves 'no labour and no pain' can only

36   Hartouni, *Cultural Conceptions*, 34.
37   Hartouni, *Cultural Conceptions*, 34.
38   Michelle Stanworth, ed., *Reproductive Technologies: Gender, Motherhood and Medicine*, Minneapolis: University of Minnesota Press, 1987, 26–7.
39   Stanworth, *Reproductive Technologies*, 26–7.
40   Stanworth, *Reproductive Technologies*, 26–7.
41   Stanworth, *Reproductive Technologies*, 26–7.

normalize the experience of men, who cannot experience reproductive labour, and exclude women's unique embodied subjectivities.[42]

Finally, Laura Woliver draws attention to the absence of the mother's contribution in the report of the 1978 birth of Louise Brown, the first so-called 'test tube' baby. The progenitors of the piece are clearly the doctors: 'After many years of frustrating research Drs Edwards and Steptoe had succeeded in removing *an egg from an ovarian follicle*, fertilizing it in a dish, and transferring the developing zygote *to a uterus where it implanted and was brought to term*'.[43] The language and composition render women's contribution to reproduction anonymous while making the role of patriarchal medical science particular and specific. The mother is present only as body parts; the only embodied agents are the doctors. Dangerous precedents have been set in the medical/scientific literature for making women's bodies, hence women's material and epistemological contribution as reproducers, invisible.

Political

NRTs can also serve as a tool for state intervention in pregnancy putatively on the foetus's behalf. Governments are taken inside women's bodies with visualization technologies raising, for some people, a responsibility to monitor what pregnant women do with their bodies. Ronda Bessner aptly reveals the repressive effects for women of the representation of foetuses as separate entities in need of societal protection while *in utero*. In 1994 she noted that Canadian and American 'child protection law, mental health legislation and criminal law'[44] were giving way to NRTs as the key vehicle of state intervention in women's reproductive lives. Citing numerous Canadian cases, she concludes that Children's Aid Societies in several provinces have applied to the courts for an order that the foetus in question is a 'child in need of protection' under the respective child welfare legislation.[45] In a new US study spanning four decades and 44 states, authors Lynn Paltrow and Jeanne Flavin found widespread denial of pregnant women's civil and political rights. They attribute such treatment to the empowerment of state actors by 'personhood measures' to 'treat fertilised eggs, embryos and foetuses as completely

---

42 Stanworth, *Reproductive Technologies*, 25–6.

43 John Robertson, 'Embryos, Families, and Procreative Liberty: The Legal Structure of the New Reproduction', *Southern California Law Review* 59:5 (1986) cited in Laura Woliver, 'The Influence of Technology on the Politics of Motherhood: An Overview of the United States', *Women's Studies International Forum* 14:5 (1991): 86. Emphasis added.

44 Ronda Bessner, 'State Intervention in Pregnancy', in *Misconceptions*, ed. Gwynne Basen, Margrit Eichler and Abby Lippman, Ontario: Voyageur Publishing, 1994, 170.

45 For example, *Re Children's Aid Society of the City of Belleville*; *Re A (in utero)* in Bessner, 'State Intervention in Pregnancy', 171 and 174. See also The Canadian Law Reform Commission's report, *Crimes Against the Fetus*: *Working Paper 58*, Department of Justice, Canada, 1989.

legally separate from the pregnant women'.[46] For example, in January 2013 Maria Guerra of Tennessee was charged with 'child endangerment and driving under the influence after she was found to be four months pregnant, even though her blood level was under the legal limit'. In addition, in an ongoing case starting in 2012, 'prosecutors in Indiana classified the failed suicide attempt of Chinese-born Bei Bei Shai, as the murder of her foetus'.[47]

Cynthia Daniels traces the history of the criminalization of pregnant women in the US back to the 1980s when '[t]he prosecution of pregnant women for fetal neglect and abuse first emerged'.[48] She cites a number of cases in which mothers-to-be have been convicted of 'criminal child neglect' (*Cornelia Whitner v. State of South Carolina* 1996), 'attempted murder of her fetus' (*State of Wisconsin v. Deborah Zimmerman* 1996), and 'endangering the welfare of a child' (Chesterfield, New Hampshire) for drug or alcohol use while pregnant. Daniels notes that as of the late nineties, most of the cases had been brought against African-American women[49] but this conclusion is reiterated in the recent report which found both that the majority of women deprived of physical liberties on the basis of their pregnancy were economically disadvantaged, and that African American women in particular were over-represented.[50]

Furthermore, disembodiment of reproduction with NRTs can heighten already existing inequalities among women in reproductive arrangements such as 'surrogacy' and egg donation. Many feminists argue that the putative benefits of NRT will not be evenly applied. Diana Taylor writes: '[p]oor women and women of color are prime targets for what has come to be known as "pure" surrogacy, an arrangement in which the woman does not provide the egg, but "only" the womb'.[51] The 'choices' women (and men) make to donate or sell body parts depend on the social structure that frames those choices, including race and class. An example is the case of Anna Johnson, who became a representative of the

46   Lynn Paltrow, quoted in Karen McVeigh, 'Study finds Widespread "Criminalization of Pregnancy" in US Institutions', *The Guardian*, 15 January 2013.

47   McVeigh, 'Study finds Widespread "Criminalization of Pregnancy" in US Institutions'.

48   Cynthia Daniels, 'Between Fathers and Fetuses: The Social Construction of Male Reproduction and the Politics of Fetal Harm', *Signs: Journal of Women in Culture and Society* 22:3 (1997): 584.

49   Daniels, 'Between Fathers and Fetuses'.

50   Lynn M. Paltrow and Jeanne Flavin, 'Arrests of and Forced Interventions on Pregnant Women in the United States, 1973–2005: Implications for Women's Legal Status and Public Health', *Journal of Health Politics, Police and Law* (2013): 299–343.

51   Dianna Taylor, 'Redefining Motherhood through Technologies and Sexualities', in *The Politics of Motherhood: Activist Voices from Left to Right*, ed. Alexis Jetter, Annelise Orleck and Diana Taylor, Hanover, NH: University Press of New England, 1997, 287. See also Sandel's BBC Reith Lecture transcripts for 'A New Citizenship', 2009; Stephanie Nolen, 'Desperate Mothers Fuel India's "baby factories"', *The Globe and Mail*, 13 February 2009.

kind of 'pure' or gestational surrogacy mentioned above, in the most publicized surrogacy case since Baby M (1988). In the California case of *Johnson v. Calvert* (1990), Johnson (a Black woman) became the gestational mother to the embryo of Mark and Crispina Calvert (a Caucasian man and his Asian-American wife). What distinguished this case from the Baby M case was the court's decision to uphold the surrogacy contract by denying Johnson parental privileges/rights to the child she gave birth to on the basis that she was not genetically related. In the Baby M case, the surrogate mother had donated her egg and was eventually considered biologically related to the child she carried. I do not intend to downplay the extreme difficulty entailed in achieving that result but to highlight the outcome.[52] The significance of *Johnson v. Calvert* surrounds the judge's likening of the gestational surrogate's role to that of a foster parent 'providing care, protection, and nurture during the period of time that the natural mother, Crispina Calvert, was unable to care for the child [since Calvert had had a hysterectomy]'.[53] For the first time a distinction was drawn between genetic and gestational motherhood, which significantly complicates the notion of 'biological'.

A key aspect of the new model of birth appropriation, expressed as NRTs, is that it not only allows men to become 'mothers' (metaphorically, literally, and in terms of celebrating male creativity by making female procreativity invisible) but with NRTs some women can become fathers. Some high-profile surrogacy cases reveal the sort of masculinization of women's reproductive consciousness and legal appropriation that occurs when some women become egg donors, uterus renters, and so on while others receive their child without the labour of pregnancy or birthing.[54] The Johnson case is particularly apt because it highlights changing conceptions of motherhood that reflect the new form of birth appropriation by modelling women's material processes of reproduction on men's. It most clearly represents the new masculinization of motherhood. Johnson v. Calvert (1990) represents the patriarchal devaluation of that part of reproduction that remains

---

52   In the Baby M case, the Judge initially characterized the donor and surrogate mother in such disparaging terms that she was socially segregated from her child and denied custody. The initial ruling was appealed and she won joint custody with the sperm donor.

53   'Calif. Judge Speaks On Issue of Surrogacy', *National Law Journal*, 5 (November 1990).

54   Janice Raymond, *Women as Wombs: Reproductive Technologies and the Battle over Women's Freedom*. San Francisco: Harper, 1993; Ruth Colker, *Pregnant Men: Practice, Theory, and the Law*. Bloomington: Indiana University Press, 1994; Bessner, 'State Intervention in Pregnancy'; Lisa Mitchell, 'The Routinization of the Other: Ultrasound, Women and the Fetus' in *Misconceptions: The Social Construction of Choice and the New Reproductive and Genetic Technologies*, Vol. 2, ed. Gwynne Basen, Margrit Eichler and Abby Lippman. Prescott, Ontario: Voyageur Publishing, 1994; Annette Burfoot, 'In-Appropriation – A Critique of "Proceed with Care: Final Report of the Royal Commission on New Reproductive Technologies"', *Women's Studies International Forum* 18:4 (1995): 499–506.

external to male experience: gestation or pregnancy. It is no surprise, then, that the genetic rather than gestational mother is privileged in law.

Alta Charo, a law professor at the University of Wisconsin, argues regarding *Johnson v. Calvert* that, 'the reality is this child has two biological mothers'.[55] The court's only woman, Justice Joyce Kennard wrote that '[a pregnant woman] is more than a mere container or breeding animal'. Hearkening back to O'Brien's analysis of reproduction she writes: 'she is the *conscious agent of creation* no less than the genetic mother, and her humanity is implicated on a deep level'.[56] More specifically, she defends the gestational mother's role and embodied motherhood, as I do.[57] Birth appropriation as a role reversal was evident in ancient Greek 'scientific' beliefs in the homunculus (or whole, 'little man' as the male contribution) in sexual reproduction. These were represented in recurrent, popular narrative themes such as in Aeschylus' *Orestes Trilogy* where it is announced that the true parent is the father, while the mother is mere nurse to his seed. Similarly, women's reproductive function in a time of the disembodiment of conception becomes more completely misaligned or distorted once interpreted through the lens of patriarchal hegemony.

At the same time, the disembodiment of reproductive process allowed by NRTs also allows men to have a more active role in reproduction, potentially equalizing the reproductive workload and bringing about a shift in reproductive roles and practices.[58] In an ideal world, women would no longer shoulder all the reproductive burden in the biological or social sense. That was what Shulamith Firestone hoped for, and what Zillah Eisenstein argues for less concretely. Eisenstein argues that women are subjugated by the naturalization of women's primary role in childrearing. She explores the liberal conflation of child-bearing and child-rearing as a particularly modern conceptualization of women's reproductive 'nature'. If women can be liberated from their role as childrearers (if not as childbearers) then they can experience their bodies as more empowering than disempowering. 'Power reflects the activity of trying to limit choices. The priorities of patriarchy are to keep the choices limited for women so that their role as mother remains primary'.[59] According to this argument, NRTs by providing more choice for some women can be seen as empowering, not just as tools of patriarchal power.

---

55   Cited in Mark Hansen, 'Surrogacy Contract Upheld: Calif. Supreme Court says such agreements don't violate public policy', *American Bar Association Journal*, August 1993.

56   Mark Hansen, 'Surrogacy Contract Upheld'. Emphasis added.

57   Arditti, 'Commercializing Motherhood', 327–8.

58   For one clear example, see Rebecca Bennett, 'Is Reproduction Women's Business? How Should We Regulate Regarding Stored Embryos, Posthumous Pregnancy, Ectogenesis and Male Pregnancy?', *Studies in Ethics, Law, and Technology* 2:3 (2008).

59   Zillah Eisenstein, *The Radical Future of Liberal Feminism*, Boston: Northeastern University Press, 1981, 16.

Conclusion, or The Paradox (of Disembodied) Reproduction

NRTs in certain legal and cultural contexts could enable us to transcend current prejudices: '[t]echnology could free women from the biological limitations of age and compulsory heterosexuality, while revamped social institutions could extend child care and educational services to all children'.[60] With NRTs, it is possible for women to have better control over their reproductive lives, undermining sex/gender inequities by making reproduction a genuine choice and 'family planning' more than a marketed slogan. The producers of NRTs cater to a new demographic of educated, career-oriented, middle-class women who are marrying later (if at all) and who have put off reproduction until later in life. In the last fifteen years there has been a sharp rise in the number of first births for women in their thirties and forties in Europe, Australia, the USA, and Canada.[61] This shift has been reflected in a spate of articles in popular magazines including *Elle Canada,* which has dubbed the situation of thirty-something women without children the 'Paula Pan syndrome', reflecting cultural assumptions about the natural (read inevitable) role of females.[62] 'Egg banks' (like sperm banks except that depositors and clients are the same) provide an expensive service for women to freeze their eggs while young so as to reproduce later.

Many herald NRTs for enabling women who are infertile, lesbians, and women with disabilities, for example, to become genetic parents without sexual reproduction (for example, the artificial womb has been marketed for cancer patients who have had hysterectomies and other involuntarily 'infertile' women). Some members of these groups take advantage of the technologies, leading to demographic changes such as the 'gaybie boom', a shorthand used by Liz Galst and Joan Hilty to explain the situation in the US since the mid-1980s in which 'lesbians began having children together as couples' rather than incorporating children from previous heterosexual couplings.[63] Family forms in the West are thus changing, as are laws. Canada's Act Concerning Assisted Reproductive Technologies and

---

60   Taylor, 'Redefining Motherhood through Technologies and Sexualities', 285.

61   Neil Seeman, 'Birth Rate Ticks, Media Roars', *Canstats Bulletins,* 12 August 2003; Ellise Pierce, Julie Scelfo and Karen Springen, 'Should You Have Your Baby Now?' *Newsweek,* 13 August 2001, 40–48; Rebecca Kippen, 'The Rise of the Older Mother', *People and Place* 14:3 (2006); Siv Gustafsson, 'Having Kids Later. Economic Analyses for Industrialized Countries', *Review of Economics of the Household* 3 (2005): 5–16.

62   Melanie Baillairge, 'Paula Pan Syndrome: A thirtysomething wonders if you have to be a mom to really feel like a woman'. *Elle Canada,* May 2002, 73. Also see Debora L. Spar, *The Baby Business: How Money, Science, and Politics Drive the Commerce of Conception,* Boston: Harvard Business School Press, 2006, where, besides arguing that the market to increase assisted conception costs does not behave at all as with normal business markets, there is relevant information on women 'choosing' to bank their eggs for later reproduction in order to establish careers.

63   Liz Galst and Joan Hilty, 'Lesbians with Strollers: The Gaybie Boom on Wheels', *Ms.* Spring 2003: 17; See also Amy Agigian, *Baby Steps,* Middletown, CT: Wesleyan

Related Research (2004), theoretically protects the equal extension of NRTs to all regardless of sexual orientation or marital status. However, while the 'infertile' are the primary intended market (and justification) for NRTs there are numerous cases which reveal that many infertility clinics refuse services to lesbians, disabled and even unmarried women.[64] In Canada the 1993 Royal Commission on New Reproductive Technologies found that fertility services were routinely refused to women who were single, lesbian, or disabled.[65] In Australia debate has raged about whether or not single women and lesbians who are believed to suffer from 'psychological infertility' should be eligible for the procedures since they are, in theory, biologically capable of reproducing without the technologies.[66] Some members of the University of Washington's infertility clinic objected to offering services to single women and lesbian couples 'on moral and religious grounds'.[67] Similarly the Warnock Report led to legislation in the UK that initially restricted all reproductive technologies, including artificial insemination, to 'stable, heterosexual couples'. Arditti also notes that in the US the only infertile women who are cared for are those who have the privilege or the health insurance to pay for techno-medical reproductive interventions. But, '[t]his is ironic, since black women, for instance, have an infertility rate one and one-half times higher than that of white women, and childlessness, for sociocultural reasons, can be a particularly devastating experience to a poor woman or a woman of color'.[68]

But times change, and the complex and dynamic exchange of social phenomena and legislation also offers room for progressive measures for women as potential reproducers. Disembodying technologies can be, and are, employed in the service of feminist goals. The technologically assisted possibility of having children for previously marginalized reproductive agents is an instance of the creative use of both social/technological and legal contexts by such actors, and a liberating influence. For example, in New Zealand, Mike Legge, Ruth Fitzgerald and Nicole Frank argue 'that new social behaviour (i.e. new understandings of "family", particularly the increasing public recognition of same-sex parenting) has produced new ART legislation'.[69] Examining case law involving ART (or NRTs as I have

University Press, 2004 and Rachel Epstein, *Who's Your Daddy? And Other Writings on Queer Parenting*, 1st edn, Toronto: Sumach Press, 2009.

64   For example, 'approximately 60 per cent of the Royal Commission report's 293 recommendations deal with the prevention of infertility and the treatments that are used to overcome it', *Proceed With Care:* Government Services Canada, 1993, 17.

65   *Proceed With Care*, Government Services Canada, 1993.

66   Gabrielle Costa, 'Backdown on "Psychological Infertility"', *The Age*, 21 November 2001.

67   Warren King and Carol M. Ostrum, 'Clinic split over fertility help for single women, lesbians', *The Las Vegas Review-Journal* (via *Seattle Times*), 12 November 1993.

68   Arditti, 'Commercializing Motherhood', 323.

69   M. Legge, R. Fitzgerald and N. Frank, 'A Retrospective Study of New Zealand Case Law involving Assisted Reproduction Technology and the Social Recognition of "New" Family', *Human Reproduction* 22:1 (2007): 17–25.

referred to them) leading up to the 2004 Human Assisted Reproduction (HART) Act they conclude there's been a social recognition of the 'new' family based on same-sex parenting, and that the use of ARTs recognizes the social reality of extended family networks that blend social as well as biological bonds. In particular they use one outcome of the Act, the national register of ART donors, donor offspring and donor siblings, to demonstrate how ART has changed contemporary New Zealand notions of family in a progressive way. The HART registry is run by the Department of Internal Affairs (administered by the Registrar General for Births, Deaths and Marriages) and is mandated to provide 'a comprehensive information-keeping regime to ensure that people born from donated embryos or donated cells can find out about their genetic origins'.[70] As of 22 August 2005, it has been mandatory for the information of all donors, donor offspring, donor offspring guardians and donor offspring siblings to be recorded and maintained.

In short, before the 2004 legislation, there was no legal recognition of the extended (beyond nuclear) family that was an outcome of routine use of the assisted reproductive technologies. The legislation in 2004, however, especially because of the register, provided legal recognition of the combined biological and social parentage of families not exclusive to, but often created by the new technology. In specific, in New Zealand, citizens have up to two mothers and two fathers legally recognized, largely because the register uses gender neutral titles like 'donors' and 'offspring' rather than 'parents' which, Legge et al. argue, is limiting in the new context of combined families, and same-sex couples.[71]

Furthermore, on the conceptual level, NRTs can indicate implicit heteronormativity in feminist theory, as Petra Nordqvist persuasively identifies in feminist critiques.[72] Investigating key ethnographic studies on NRTs she found that heterosexuality remains 'foundational to, and yet invisible within, this feminist research into reproductive technologies'.[73] Furthermore, disability theorist Susan Wendell cautions us against romanticizing embodiment as uniformly and always welcomed, especially during times of chronic pain for example. Similarly, political scientist Candace Johnson examines the political, socially situated nature of the call for 'natural' non-technologically mediated forms of reproduction. As one point of caution, they reveal privilege not shared by all, as Johnson argues that for women of lower socio-economic status the absence of certain routine technologies is of more concern than unwanted 'unnatural' technological intervention in their reproductive processes as they can appear in feminist critiques of NRTs.[74]

---

70   Legge et al., 'A Retrospective Study', 23.

71   Legge et al., 'A Retrospective Study', 23.

72   Petra Nordqvist, 'Feminist Heterosexual Imaginaries of Reproduction: Lesbian Conception in Feminist Studies of Reproductive Technologies, *Feminist Theory* 9:3 (2008): 273–92.

73   Nordqvist, 'Feminist Heterosexual Imaginaries of Reproduction', 273.

74   Candace Johnson, 'The Political 'Nature' of Childbirth and Pregnancy', *Canadian Journal of Political Science* 41:4 (2008): 889–913.

In the final analysis it is important to re-centre focus on 'the socio-legal forces that control technology' because '[t]echnology is a means to an end'[75] which calls for a focus on the cultural and ideological context of its development and use. For instance, a forced tubal litigation in rural India bears little resemblance to a sought out sterilization procedure in an affluent Western suburb. However, the overarching concern is the continuing epistemology of dualism (mind versus body) that enables NRTs to offer 'control' at the cost of disembodiment, or fragmentation of embodied corporeality, and what this excludes. Mainstream reproductive discourse, and feminist theories of reproduction that offer women better lives via 'control' over their reproductive bodies, beg the question: what notion of liberation underlies 'better lives' based on NRTs. I am sympathetic to the work of Wendi Hadd and other critical analyses of the discourses that equate power and control over physiology (including embodied reproduction). In particular, I agree that the association of power with control over nature is too steeped in uncritical patriarchal scientific models to be uncritically adopted by feminists. The very language of 'control' over women's reproduction exposes a partial perspective that may distort issues of embodiment which are of fundamental importance to feminism. Wendell (1988) reminds us that bodies are not only sources of pleasure to be simply 'reclaimed' for women, and debunks the myth of western medicine that we can 'control' our bodies.

---

75   Hadd, 'A Womb with a View', 171.

PART II
Feminism and New Reproductive Technologies

Introduction to Part II

In Part II, I argue that women's reproductive consciousnesses are shaped on a number of levels by the birth appropriative elements of the Western canon, and especially along the lines of the patriarchal dualism we've been exploring. Feminists have theorized and resisted different politically entrenched sex/gender regimes, developing their own ideologies and strategies with regard to the relationships between nature and convention. In terms of general trends in feminist thinking (which are often underpinned by liberal/mainstream feminist ideas), the 'first wave' in the Anglo-American feminist movement was primarily maternalist in orientation, drawing on patriarchal stereotypes about women's superior 'natural' morality to gain women's civil and political rights. The 'second wave' was largely socially constructionist, striving to reveal the conventional nature of patriarchal systems in order to deconstruct them. But now women's reproductive consciousnesses are increasingly assimilated into androcentric canonical paradigms because of NRTs and erosion of the material base of women's sex/gender differences from men. The birth appropriation of the canon is no longer just ideological, but also material. Can feminists and women subvert patriarchal dualism (e.g. masculinized political realm/feminized natural realm) at the heart of varying sex/gender regimes upheld by states? Some feminists have merely incorporated this dualism in fleeing from the 'natural' body by using NRTs, or in embracing the 'natural' body and fleeing NRTs; others are more equivocal about the 'nature' of the body.

Feminists approach the disembodiment of women's reproductive processes wrought by NRTs in at least three categorical ways: *resistance* to, *embrace* of, and *equivocal* regarding the technologies. In the next two chapters I evaluate each position on the basis of its ability to transcend patriarchal dualism in its often underlying treatment of the man/technology over woman/nature value binary in modern Western societies. In Chapter 4, both the resisting feminists and embracing feminists reassert patriarchal dualism, fostering an essentialized notion of 'woman' associated with 'nature' on the basis of her reproductive functions. That is, the resisting and embracing feminists are remnants of traditions in which the body is viewed as 'naturally' oppressive or liberating, associated with the premodern conflation of the realms of biology and society, for example, in Robert Filmer's notion of the divine right of kings which erased the division between natural, paternal authority and governmental power. Embracers, however, come from a long line of postmodern thinking about the necessary and possible transcendence of the body's 'natural' boundaries via cyberspace and other creative reconfigurations. These existentialist impulses are characterized by what is considered 'the body's' malleability to social forces and reconstructions, in combination with a sense of 'the body' as restricting rather than enabling.

In Chapter 3, equivocal feminists, as the name suggests, incorporate elements of both the embracing and resisting feminist responses, and while they tend to adopt a social constructionist view of 'the body', like Hobbes, they perceive 'the body' (as in our biological roots) as neither naturally oppressive, nor necessarily liberating. It is not definitely a liability, though sex/gender differences are socially significant, and matter in terms of power and politics, especially because of reproduction.

Chapter 2
Resistors and Embracers

The complexity of embodied reproductive experiences may not be reduced to one or the other 'universal' experience of binary normative sex, but it remains severely restricted by what it means to be a man or a woman in Western cultures. It is more than empty liberal rhetoric when new reproductive technology (NRT) policies like in Canada and New Zealand, name women as especially implicated in, and affected by, their uses. Therefore, since the ethics and politics of NRTs demands it of women, I have argued for a rapprochement with Mary O'Brien's focus on reproduction as part of the 'post-constructionist' turn – not as biologically determined but firmly rooted in the enduring dialectic of sex/gender.[1]

Part of the value of O'Brien's theory of male and female reproductive consciousnesses is its antidote to the current fragmentation of women's identities, *qua* women. Unlike O'Brien, however, we must acknowledge that part of this fragmentation is women's diverse experiences of their reproductive capacity. Her perspective over privileges the shared dimensions of women's corporeality and consciousness, whereas much current feminist theorizing of the body endlessly fragments women's experiences, but we must have both shared and diverse experiences for viable feminist movements.[2] 'Reproductive consciousness' is significantly more complicated than O'Brien's singular phrasing suggests. 'Feminine reproductive consciousness' does not simply involve the corporeal capacity to be pregnant and give birth (though it does include it); or just the considerably fraught 'choice' to *not* birth that contraceptive technology offered. Greater technological and social intervention provides for the 'choice' to specify what kind of children to have, and when and how. Our capacity to impose social and cultural norms on biological continuity and process has never been greater. For example, NRTs allow lesbians, gay men, and women with disabilities among others to reproduce biologically, which is a significant socio-cultural and political shift, as well as a biomedical one. Although human reproduction is not altogether disembodied, in the sense of taking place fully outside the female body as some feminist theory and literature envisioned, it is more so than ever before.[3] In such a time it is not surprising that the feminist response to NRTs has been so great and diverse.

---

1   Nina Lykke. 'The Timeliness of Post-Constructionism', *NORA – Nordic Journal of Feminist and Gender Research* 18:2 (June 2010): 131–6.

2   Vanaja Dhruvarajan and Jill Vickers, eds, *Gender, Race, and Nation: A Global Perspective*, Toronto: University of Toronto Press, 2002.

3   Shulamith Firestone, *The Dialectic of Sex: The Case for Feminist Revolution*, New York: Quill William Morrow, 1970; Marge Piercy, *Woman on the Edge of Time*, New York: Ballantine Books, 1976.

This chapter explores two seemingly oppositional forms of feminist discourse that have emerged in response to NRTs since the 1980s, representing the disembodying of reproductive processes, and analyses the notion of liberation which underlies each. *Resistance* feminism and *embracing* feminism are each evaluated on the basis of its ability to transcend patriarchal dualism and reveal birth appropriation in various guises by exploring how each draws on or subverts the man/technology over woman/nature value dualism. I draw attention to feminists' varying discursive responses to technoscience-enabled *ex vivo* procreation. Feminists who embrace the technology and are rooted in the radical materialist feminist manifesto of Shulamith Firestone respond quite differently from the feminists who resist NRTs and are inspired by the radical and eco-feminist principles of such thinkers as Germaine Greer and Vandana Shiva. Feminist resistors who were most active during roughly 1984–1991 constitute a 'first phase' of feminist critique of NRTs to adopt Charis Thompson's useful framing. The key distinction is between this first phase which is largely, though not wholly, defined by explicit resistance to NRTs and a 'second phase' (roughly 1992–2001) coinciding with the linguistic turn in social science of the late 1980s/ early 1990s and influenced by it. With regard to the essentialism/constructionism debate, the first resistance phase is often characterized by an essentialized view of motherhood (variously valorized or denigrated) and the second by an official opposition to the former's 'essentialism'.

I am particularly interested in the different discursive strategies feminists use regarding 'new' reproductive technologies as they are circumscribed within the residual framework of 'old' reproductive technology (abortion). Ultimately all feminists approach NRTs with the belief that women must be able to 'control' their own reproduction, but they differ in their definitions of such control.[4] Their ideas are inevitably framed by the discourse of 'choice' which has dominated Western feminist abortion debates. Also, the different but converging theoretical roots of various feminist responses to disembodiment are important indicators of possible directions for overcoming the constructionist/essentialist impasse in 'post-constructionist' feminisms.

Resistance Feminism

Resistance feminists, who argue against new reproductive technologies, believe there is something powerful about women's 'natural' (non-technologically mediated) reproductive bodies that is lost with NRTs. Since few reject contraceptive

---

4   For a history of competing feminist uses of 'control', see Bette Vanderwater, 'Meanings and Strategies of Reproductive Control: Current Feminist Approaches to Reproductive Technology', *Issues in Reproductive and Genetic Engineering* 5:3 (1992): 215–30; Rosalind Pollack Petchesky, 'Reproductive Freedom: Beyond "a woman's right to choose"', *Signs – The Journal of Women in Culture and Society* 5 (Summer 1980): 661–85.

technology on the same basis, this position leads to a fundamental contradiction in their discourse, and in feminist discourse more generally concerning the technological mediation of reproduction. The resistors recognize in women's sex/ reproduction both a source of vulnerability in patriarchal cultures, and also one of power provided *women control it*. They reject NRTs because they see them as an extension of the patriarchal desire to control nature and women, rooted in men's reproductive alienation from nature since their role ends in ejaculation, rather than birth. Technoscience, in this framework, is a birth appropriative technology designed and used by men to overcome their reproductive alienation from nature.[5]

Similarly, most resistance feminists believe that, even if women controlled NRTs, they could not 'purify the technology out of its political base'.[6] Furthermore, through discourse analysis about NRTs, resistance feminists reveal the sociopolitical inequalities in which they are rooted, masked by various benevolent representations. They deconstruct the discourse of NRT as presenting *the* 'choice' for the infertile in light of the reality of a culture marked by power differences and control. Ultimately, resistance feminists argue that women's liberation requires their collective control over their own sexuality and reproduction (rather than individual 'choice'), and freedom from NRT as a patriarchal technology that entrenches control over women in the hands of patriarchal authorities, be they medical, scientific, capitalist, or state technocrats.

Resistance feminists begin from the premise that women's 'natural' reproductive processes are a source of (feminist) identity and empowerment that is exclusively theirs. Greer best articulates the resistance position: 'Refusing to be defined, discriminated against and disadvantaged because of our female biology should not be confused with a demand to be deprived of it'.[7] Since the emphasis is on commonality amongst women, based on the potential for pregnancy and birth rather than women's differences from each other, her use of 'women' is deemed biologically reductionist in Judith Butler's sense. Since conservative and anti-feminist arguments are rooted in the same uncritical postulation of women's 'nature' as linked to reproduction this has led to calls for political coalitions based on shared values, rather than 'biological' commonalities.

The underlying assumption of such expressions of women's resistance and power is that to alter women's bodies (their 'nature' in a sense), as NRTs do, is to weaken or undermine women. NRTs' intervention in women's bodies and natural reproductive processes somehow threatens all women's power, autonomy and control over their bodies. Implicitly associating women with their biology is the basis of the main critique of the resistance position. They reify patriarchal dualism while arguing

---

5   This womb-envy argument is the foundation of the political theory of feminists such as Mary O'Brien (*The Politics of Reproduction; Reproducing the World*); and Carole Pateman (*The Sexual Contract* and 'The Fraternal Social Contract').

6   Robyn Rowland, *Living Laboratories: Women and Reproductive Technology*, London: Lime Tree, 1992, 292.

7   Germaine Greer, *The Whole Woman*, Toronto: Doubleday, 1999, 325.

against it, which is further highlighted in the belief that technology is a continuation of patriarchal science that destroys nature, and by association, women.

The ecofeminism at the core of the resistance argument draws explicitly from this man/technology, and woman/nature analogy regarding NRTs. The writing of Shiva and Maria Mies are the best examples.[8] Irene Diamond reinforces the women-nature connection by linking environmental degradation to infertility and reproductive problems.[9] This theme of fertility/infertility and birth defects as an indicator of the condition of the natural world recurs in feminist and mainstream science fiction. Margaret Atwood's *The Handmaid's Tale*, is predicated upon a dystopic future society of reproductive fundamentalism, partly because pollution has caused mass infertility and a one-in-four chance of giving birth to a deformed child. The handmaidens are the fertile women, 'wombs with two legs', who are 'naturally' inseminated surrogates for the infertile wives of rich and powerful commanders. In Gilead of Atwood's tale, women's social status is linked to their reproductive capacities. Here 'natural' maternity is valued but its rarity legitimizes a reproductive fundamentalism in which every aspect of womens' existence is monitored.

Similarly P.D. James's novel *Children of Men* betrays cultural anxieties about an infertility-driven dystopia set in England in the year 2021. Mass infertility and the grim realization that the final generation has just turned 25 create the anxious backdrop. Akin to Atwood's warning, *Children of Men* centres on the discovery of a pregnant woman after many years of global infertility and how this precious entity now needs protection. This rare occurrence makes the mother-to-be a valuable commodity with immeasurable sociopolitical, economic, and even symbolic value – but also one that faces danger on all sides. The pregnancy in James' narrative reveals the paradoxical character of the woman-nature association, especially for women who are the reproducers.

Shiva and others note that NRT further displaces the power of nature from women to male doctors through 'the relocation of knowledge and skills from the mother to the doctor'.[10] The resister's position is underscored by distrust for the Western scientific paradigms seen as based on domination of nature and of women by association.[11] This line of thought can be traced to Carolyn Merchant's *The Death of Nature*, in which modern science is depicted as the epitome of Man versus Nature (conceived as female). Merchant's comprehensive history of

---

8   Vandana Shiva, *Biopiracy: The Plunder of Nature and Knowledge*, Toronto: Between the Lines, 1999, 5.

9   Irene Diamond, *Fertile Ground: Women, Earth, and the Limits of Control*, Boston: Beacon Press, 1994, 97.

10   Shiva, *Biopiracy*, 58.

11   Gena Corea, *The Mother Machine: Reproductive Technologies from Artificial Insemination to Artificial Wombs*, New York: Harper and Row, 1985, 5. See also Patricia Spallone, *Beyond Conception: The New Politics of Reproduction*, Basingstoke: Macmillan Education Ltd, 1989, 187.

Western conceptions of nature, explains how dominant nature metaphors shifted from the more organic in pre-modern times to that of nature as machine (as epitomized in Hobbes) in the context of the scientific revolution. She concludes that the 'death of nature' coincided with the victory of a mechanistic metaphor for nature, reflecting the triumph of empirical science and development of technology to dissect 'mother nature' in various ways.

While such feminist theorists describe a patriarchal technoscientific paradigm rooted in ancient conceptions of women/nature, as well as Enlightenment science (as Merchant reveals), the 'new' reproductive technologies are tools within a continuing paradigm. What's new about them is that they are highly technological, even if they do partake of a well-established androcentric scientific worldview. NRTs are also institutionally entrenched and commercialized, so further from feminist access, and require the state to regulate and protect women. They may eventually allow men to create babies, rather than simply allow women not to have them, which could destabilize sexist sex/gender roles, but only where the material and social relations of reproduction are radically altered.[12] Also, with NRTs, physical disembodiment is greater, which further entrenches and universalizes patriarchal epistemologies.

The resistors' position forms part of an ongoing and longstanding feminist debate about the role of a patriarchal biomedical science in pathologizing women's sex/gender difference throughout history. Cecilia Asberg considers feminist technoscience studies an outgrowth of 'health activist movements, early feminist critiques of science and women's engagement with medical, ecological and scientific issues'; an especially noteworthy example being the globally renowned feminist self-help text *Our Bodies, Ourselves* first produced by the Boston Women's Health Book Collective in 1971.[13] Similarly Thompson writes 'feminist writings that were critical of reproductive technologies grew out of and in turn developed several themes that were core parts of second wave feminist scholarship on science, medicine, child-birth, and reproductive rights'.[14] Women's selfhood (and subjectivity) was impossible to dissociate from their embodiment or, put differently, the body was intrinsic to the self in that radical period.

Resistance feminists analyse NRTs as extensions of an inherently patriarchal science that encompasses both ways of knowing as well as technological apparatuses. Most importantly, science's two dimensions are considered mutually supportive; science creates cultural contexts for the reception of new technologies like NRT. Patricia Spallone, for example, tried to 'show how technology redefines the meaning of reproduction in society to the detriment of women, how technology

---

12   Petchesky, 'Reproductive Freedom'.

13   Celia Asberg, 'Enter Cyborg: Tracing the Historiography and Ontological Turn of Feminist Technoscience studies', *International Journal of Feminist Technoscience* 1:1 (2010): 11.

14   Charis Thompson, *Making Parents: The Ontological Choreography of Reproductive Technologies*, USA: Massachusetts Institute of Technology Press, 2005, 57.

sets a repressive ethic of reproduction, and in turn how repressive social relations provide the conditions for the technologies to happen'.[15]

Resistance feminists argue that displacement of women's 'natural' embodied power by a patriarchal scientific establishment requires disembodiment of women, accomplished by interrupting the woman-nature connection symbolically and literally. With NRTs this is done by radical reconceptualization of modern Western conceptions of nature and culture and the relationship between the two; and the reduction of women to body parts, mere matter to be manipulated by 'techno-docs'.[16] These practices are simultaneous and mutually reinforcing and contribute to the representation of man-the-scientist as father, cue Mary Shelley's Frankenstein.

Merete Lie asserts a central role for science in new understandings about what 'natural' reproduction is. This includes the understanding of reproduction as natural, biological processes and of the body as a product of nature'.[17] These conceptual distinctions are profoundly gendered, and women's historic and psycho-socially deep rooted associations with nature and the body make this shift particularly pronounced for them. According to Lie, NRTs sever the woman-nature connection via motherhood. Men have appropriated women's unique role in reproduction not just in discourse, but also in its material processes. 'An implicit message of the new stories of procreation is that science has gained insight into the totality of the process. Symbolically, woman is no longer 'the creator of children' in accordance with the cultural theory of *matrigenesis*, but rather one of several participants in a process'.[18] Paradoxically, the mother is ousted and usurped by scientific rationale in a culture built upon faith in scientific expertise, but also 'freed' from her body, if not from its consequences.

For resistance feminists, scientific epistemology is synonymous with the dissection of women by association with nature, in the name of a patriarchally defined 'progress'. Spallone argues that women become the essential 'raw materials of research' required for experimentation and creation of human life.[19] For example, because conception occurs outside the womb with NRTs, women's eggs need to be donated in an arrangement like sperm donation and some would argue women become the site of harmful medical experimentation. Annette Burfoot and others have written about the significance of this new reproductive disembodiment for women in terms of it masculinizing their reproductive consciousness as I do here.[20]

Resistance feminists argue that foetal visualization technologies, like sonograms, literally take women out of the picture and make embryos/foetuses

---

    15 Spallone, *Beyond Conception*, 4.
    16 Merete Lie, 'Science as Father? Sex and Gender in the Age of Reproductive Technologies', *The European Journal of Women's Studies* 9:4 (2002).
    17 Lie, 'Science as Father?', 383.
    18 Lie, 'Science as Father?', 393–394; Greer, *The Whole Woman*, 82.
    19 Spallone, *Beyond Conception*, 6.
    20 Annette Burfoot, 'In-Appropriation'.

seem independent. Foetal visualization literally enables a reproductive refocus on a previously invisible entity, the foetus, which, as many resistance feminists have documented, through technology becomes a liberal rights-bearing individual who may threaten its mother's autonomy, integrity, and rights. This dissection allows patriarchal interests to intervene more in women's bodies. Feminists have written widely about the 'rollback effects' of foetal visualization technologies, or ultrasound, for women's rights.[21] In legal and popular contexts, new visualizing technologies and communication technologies provide fresh fodder for anti-abortion activists resulting in the imposition of an antagonistic relationship between mother and foetus in a liberal rights framework. Many feminists link the development of NRTs to the proliferation of court cases related to the monitoring and restriction of every aspect of women's behaviour while pregnant.[22]

Analysing reproductive discourse since the advent of NRTs provides resistance feminists with much evidence of women's disembodiment. Literary as well as visual texts illustrate how NRTs disembody women and consequently present opportunities for the usurpation of women's reproductive significance by technoscientists. Regarding foetal visualization technology, Lisa Mitchell clarifies the connection: 'ultrasound transforms pregnant women from embodied, thinking, and knowledgeable individuals into "maternal environments", or tissue that may or may not yield a clear ultrasound image'.[23] Similarly, in her analysis of medical discourse in US government publications Spallone curiously found 'there are no women mentioned as the subject of human reproduction. [T]here are body parts and biological processes but there are no women as whole human beings'.[24] Resistance feminists recognize that medicalization of birth/reproduction is hardly new, but they believe conceptive technologies and techniques of NRTs further threaten women's reproductive autonomy.

---

21 For example Rosalind Petchesky, 'Foetal Images: The Power of Visual Culture in the Politics of Reproduction', in *Reproductive Technologies: Gender, Motherhood and Medicine*, ed. Michelle Stanworth, Minneapolis: University of Minnesota Press, 1987, 57–80; Ann Oakley, 'The History of Ultrasonography in Obstetrics', *Birth*, 13 (supplement) (1986): 5–10; Susan Squier, 'Fetal Subjects and Maternal Objects: Reproductive Technology and the New Fetal/Maternal Relation', *The Journal of Medicine and Philosophy* 21:5 (1996): 515–35; Sarah Franklin, 'Postmodern Procreation: A Cultural Account of Assisted Reproduction', in *Conceiving The New World Order: The Global Politics of Reproduction*, ed. Faye D. Ginsburg and Rayna Rapp, Berkeley: University of California Press, 1995, 323–45; and Valerie Hartouni. *Cultural Conceptions: On Reproductive Technologies and The Remaking of Life*, Minneapolis: University of Minnesota Press, 1997.

22 See Chapter 1.

23 Lisa Mitchell, *Baby's First Picture: Ultrasound and the Politics of Fetal Subjects*, Toronto: University of Toronto Press, 2001, 20; Cites also William R. Arney, *Power and the Profession of Obstetrics*, Chicago: University of Chicago Press, 1982; Ann Oakley, *The Captured Womb: A History of the Medical Care of Pregnant Women*, Oxford: Basil Blackwell, 1986; Oakley, 'The History of Ultrasonography in Obstetrics'.

24 Spallone, *Beyond Conception*, 16.

Valerie Hartouni sees the ultimate expression of women as foetus-containers in a *San Francisco Chronicle* headline that read: 'Orphan Embryos Saved'.[25] This, together with other headlines such as 'Brain Dead Mother Has Her Baby', she explains, highlights cultural beliefs that motherhood is a passive process requiring little agency or even sentience on the part of women; embryos are autonomous agents with a right to life before being born. The other side of this misconception is the notion that techno-medical intervention is welcomed, *natural*, and perhaps even *necessary* to sustain life.[26] As Pamela Moore, Sarah Franklin and others have noted, this is part of the 'naturalization of reproductive technology' by its presentation as an ordinary part of women's lives, drawing more women into habitual use of NRTs, just as they were persuaded they needed doctors and hospitals to give birth.[27]

Gena Corea demonstrates the depth of resistor's distrust of Western medicine when she claims that a form of reproductive prostitution that also commodifies parts of women's bodies, modelled on sexual prostitution will also be the result of the normalization of NRTs.[28] Some would argue that her fears were substantiated with the reality of reproductive tourism globally, and cross-class surrogacy within national boundaries. Like Mies and other resistance feminists, Corea distrusts a medical and scientific establishment with a history of 'abusing' women, and others, for material profit and patriarchal values.

Infertility and 'Choice'

Resistance feminists reject the view that NRTs are simply about providing 'choice' for infertile women and men. Rather, they see NRTs as extending patriarchal control over female reproduction, exploiting it for power and profit. Furthermore, they believe NRTs are about social control under the guise of individual choice, i.e. they serve to mask industrial/social problems with therapy for infertile individuals. They are wary of the NRTs discourse, partly because it partakes of a liberal rights and an inherently androcentric liberal individualist framework.[29]

---

25   Hartouni, *Cultural Conceptions*, 27.

26   Franklin, 'Postmodern Procreation'. See also Hartouni, *Cultural Conceptions*, 56–7.

27   Pamela L. Moore, 'Selling Reproduction', in *Playing Dolly: Technocultural Formations, Fantasies, and Fictions of Assisted Reproduction*, ed. E. Ann Kaplan and Susan Squier, New Brunswick: Rutgers University Press, 1999.

28   Moore, 'Selling Reproduction'.

29   For example, following Carol Pateman, '"God Hath Ordained to Man a Helper": Hobbes, Patriarchy and Conjugal Right', in *Feminist Interpretations and Political Theory*, ed. Mary Lyndon Shanley and Carole Pateman, University Park, PA: Pennsylvanian State University Press, 1991, 53–73; Carol Pateman, *The Sexual Contract*, Cambridge/Stanford: Polity/Stanford University Press, 1988; Carol Pateman, 'The Fraternal Social Contract', in *Civil Society and the State: New European Perspectives*, ed. J. Keane, London and New

Undermining the NRT discourse resistance feminists focus on collective, rather than individual, solutions to reproductive problems such as infertility, and blur the social/biological division by refusing to consider biological problems in isolation from social inequality. For example, Mies asserts that 'fertility or sterility are not just biological conditions and "diseases" but socially determined'.[30] This statement can be taken in two senses: first, that the 'epidemic' of infertility has been socially constructed; and second, that problems associated with infertility have socio-cultural origins. Resistance feminists examine both and also the notion that not having your 'own' kids is 'a problem'.

In *Misconceptions,* the editors examine '[t]he construction of infertility'.[31] They claim that despite the lack of reliable statistics on infertility in Canada, 'numbers ranging from one in six to as high as one in three couples "affected" by infertility are consistently touted by those who have a vested interest in manufacturing an "epidemic"'.[32] Resistance feminists argue that the social significance associated with infertility is recent. It is because we now believe that NRTs can 'cure' infertility that we believe it must be cured. As Lie and others have noted, infertility and fertility are designations subject to change depending on varying conceptions of the natural, which as we've seen are socially defined. For example, the Canadian Royal Commission on New Reproductive Technologies defined infertility as the lack of conception by couples co-habiting for two years without using contraception when the woman was between eighteen and forty-four, but this is not a uniform standard.[33]

Resistance feminists note that the socio-cultural and political power at the root of problems that NRT 'fixes' are masked by the 'technological fix' approach. They remind us that '[i]t is in the obvious interests of the reproductive industry to sell infertility as a growing individual problem demanding a strictly medical-technological solution', despite the considerable collective social/cultural problems that threaten reproductive health.[34] They argue that environmental pollution, unsafe workplaces, and medical practices themselves create infertility and reproductive problems that are overlooked because of the dominance of pro-

---

York: Verso, 1988, 101–27; Zillah Eisenstein, *The Radical Future of Liberal Feminism,* Boston: Northeastern University Press, 1981; and others.

30　Maria Mies, 'New Reproductive Technologies: Sexist and Racist Implications', in *Ecofeminism,* ed. Maria Mies and Vandana Shiva, Halifax, Nova Scotia: Fermwood Publications, 1993, 174–97.

31　Gwynne Basen, Margrit Eichler and Abby Lippman, eds, *Misconceptions: The Social Construction of Choice and the New Reproductive and Genetic Technologies,* Vol. 2, Prescott, Ontario: Voyageur Publishing, 1994, 13.

32　Basen, et al., *Misconceptions,* Vol. 2, p. 14.

33　Government Services Canada, *Proceed With Care: Final Report of the Royal Commission on New Reproductive Technologies,* Ottawa, Canada: Minister of Government Services Canada, 1993.

34　Heather Menzies, 'The Social Construction of Reproductive Technologies and of Choice', in Basen et al., *Misconceptions,* Vol. 2, p. 5.

technoscientific discourse in which NRTs are entrenched.[35] Similarly, postponing childbirth to pursue financial and social stability is not strictly a biological matter. In this view, NRTs become a technological fix for very real, if harder to isolate, social problems resulting from the rationalization of reproduction in line with the patriarchal development of NRTs.

Resistance feminists argue that if contemporary sexual and reproductive issues were viewed through a feminist lens, the proposed solutions would be different. For example if infertility, most often perceived as a biological problem, cannot in reality be disentwined from its sociopolitical roots, neither can its solutions. Abby Lippman, for example, analysing the 'geneticization' of both health and reproduction, provides a 'worrisome example ... in the identification of a gene associated with susceptibility to lead poisoning'.[36] This discovery detracts from the social and political causes and solution to the problem of lead poisoning which, she suggests, would most simply and cheaply entail replacing substandard housing, where lead-based paint is found with decent accommodations.[37] Similarly, when it comes to infertility related to postponement wouldn't national daycare programs, parental leave and other work-life balance promoting policies encourage reproduction before NRTs are necessary? Furthermore with the political will for, and completion of, the human genome project such genetics-centric approaches to health, reproduction, and well-being tend to dominate.[38]

NRT discourse appropriates the liberal rights framework feminists used to win abortion rights. The pro-NRTs position is pro-choice. But as Janice Raymond reminds us, '[t]o be pro-choice ... is *not* necessarily to be pro-woman'.[39] Spallone challenges the idea that NRTs innocently provide women with '[a]nother reproductive "choice"' rather than serving 'the various needs and desires of medical scientists, research scientists, and the state to further technological "progress" and to aid population control aims'.[40] Furthermore, some resistance feminists like Robyn Rowland argue that the 'infertile' have no real 'choice'; that is, in patriarchal cultures that define women by their reproductive function, infertility becomes pathology and women are pressured into embracing NRTs.[41] Finally, Barbara

---

35   Karen Messing and Gail Ouellette, 'A Prevention Oriented Approach to Reproductive Problems: Identifying Environmental Effects', in *Misconceptions: The Social Construction of Choice and the New Reproductive and Genetic Technologies*, Vol. 1, ed. Gwynne Basen, Margrit Eichler and Abby Lippman, Prescott, Ontario: Voyageur Publishing, 1993; Corea, *The Mother Machine*; Spallone, *Beyond Conception*; Diamond, *Fertile Ground*.

36   Basen et al. *Misconceptions*, Vol. 1, p. 58.

37   Basen et al. *Misconceptions*, Vol. 1, p. 59.

38   Marque-Luisa Miringoff, *The Social Costs of Genetic Welfare*, New Brunswick, New Jersey: Rutgers University Press, 1991.

39   Janice Raymond, *Women as Wombs: Reproductive Technologies and the Battle Over Women's Freedom*, San Francisco: Harper, 1993, 85.

40   Spallone, *Beyond Conception*, 2.

41   Rowland, *Living Laboratories*.

Katz Rothman wrote that what is passed off as 'choice' may mean less choice for mothers, showing how the social and cultural infrastructure that accompanies any new technology becomes the most significant aspect of technological change.[42] 'It seems that, in gaining the choice to control the quality of our children, we may be losing the choice not to control the quality'.[43] For example, the socio-cultural and historically specific perception of disability, teamed with the possibility of a genetic 'abnormality' developing into a 'disability', may preclude the possibility of refusing a test to prevent the birth of such a child. In Canada, about 97 per cent of all pregnant women now undergo at least one ultrasound scan; physicians do not have to have a woman's consent to perform the procedure.[44] In like vein it may be asked whether the 'choice' for those who postpone childbirth to establish financial and other resources will be, struggling with motherhood at a younger age without the appropriate means, or IVF?

Resistance feminists argue that if NRTs were genuinely about choice, we would first have to address the context of inequality which currently undermines it.[45] Who or what ultimately controls which choices are available? Too often, the debates are reduced to polar opposition, to those who are simply 'for or against IVF and the women who use it'.[46] Such polarization precludes discussion of NRTs' usefulness and conversely its potential detrimental effects, which diminishes real choice. Prominent pro-choice abortion activist Judy Rebick highlights that 'In a class and race-divided society, freedom of choice for one woman can mean virtual slavery for another, for example contract motherhood'; thus, protecting some women from the exploitation that NRTs will inevitably bring justifies the abrogation of some women's individual freedom of choice.[47] In addition, they believe feminist efforts should, ultimately, 'reject the equation of personhood with fertility'.[48]

Resistance feminists believe that the oppressive dimensions of womanhood and motherhood come from patriarchal and capitalist definitions of women's biology and not some biological essence of womanhood. Nonetheless some resistors call for a rethinking of the prioritization of biological over various types of social motherhood. They advocate for women's control over their own reproduction, which includes the social and political infrastructure and resources to mother without impoverishment and other socio-cultural barriers. However, there is a lingering Beauvoirian anti-natalism in resistance feminists' position. This poses a

---

42 Barbara Katz-Rothman, 'The Meanings of Choice in Reproductive Technology', in *Test-Tube Women: What Future for Motherhood?*, ed. Rita Arditti, Renate Duelli Klein and Shelley Minden, London: Pandora Press, 1984.

43 Cited in Rowland, *Living Laboratories*, 286.

44 Mitchell, *Baby's First Picture*, 5.

45 See for example Spallone, *Beyond Conception*, 65; Corea, *The Mother Machine*, 3.

46 Basen et al., *Misconceptions*, Vol. 1, pp. 13–14.

47 Judy Rebick, 'Is the Issue Choice?', in Basen et al., *Misconceptions*, Vol. 1, p. 88.

48 Rowland, *Living Laboratories*, 297.

contradiction for resisters expressed most clearly in inconsistent arguments about abortion (old reproductive technology) and NRTs.

A concern for many resistance feminists is reconciling the contradictory opposition to NRTs on the basis of choice, with their support of contraceptive technologies, also based on the language of 'choice'. As Rowland notes '"a woman's right to choose" is "a woman's right to *control*"' where abortion enables women 'to control their lives in a less than perfect world'. When it comes to conceptive technologies however, she believes that the choice to use them decreases women's reproductive control.[49] Ultimately, she defends the 'right to choose' old reproductive technology but not new reproductive technology by making it fit within an argument for control, based on the negative 'freedom from' NRTs rather than the positive 'freedom to' use them, endorsing contraceptive technologies because they offer women freedom from babies.[50] Addressing the issue of control inherent in questions of women's 'choice' in patriarchal societies, resistance feminists are embroiled in a difficult contradiction.

In resistance feminists' discourse, NRT is really about extension of patriarchal control. As Spallone notes 'removing technologies will [not] automatically give back to women control over our own bodies', invoking *The Handmaid's Tale* as a caveat.[51] For many resistance feminists this control implies that 'Like all groups who "own" a capacity such as this, women want to hold onto their exclusivity'.[52] But Raymond defends the resistance position from its distortion through the bifurcating social constructionism versus essentialism lens within feminism:

> Radical feminist opponents of the new reproductive technologies do not pit nature against technology, nor do we extol a new version of biology is destiny for women. Opposition to these technologies is based on the more political feminist perspective that women as a class have a stake in reclaiming the female body, not as female nature, but by refusing to yield control of it to men, to the fetus, to the state, and most recently to those liberals who advocate that women control our bodies by giving up control.[53]

Regarding NRTs as merely another set of tools for patriarchal control over female sexuality/reproduction and nature, they advocate rejection and a moratorium over all NRTs because they devalue women and nature, and usurp women's reproductive control.[54] In Canada, both the National Action Committee on the Status of Women (NAC) and the Feminist International Network of Resistance to Reproductive and Genetic Technologies (FINRRAGE) presented briefs to the Royal Commission on

---

49   Rowland, *Living Laboratories*, 285.
50   Raymond, *Women as Wombs*.
51   Spallone, *Beyond Conception*, 5.
52   Rowland, *Living Laboratories*, 13.
53   Raymond, *Women as Wombs*, 91.
54   Rowland, *Living Laboratories*, 13.

NRTs supporting such a moratorium in order to 'hold on to their [reproductive] exclusivity'.[55] Resistance to NRTs looks a lot like a call for re-embodiment – a defence of the body – with the undesirable consequence of a continued female/ nature association that is easily allied with neo-conservative politics.

Embracing Feminists

Feminists who advocate the use of NRTs, embracing feminists, argue that reproduction is oppressive for women and that technologies that disembody female reproductive process can liberate them.[56] Female embodiment becomes synonymous with historically-evidenced, patriarchal oppression and liberation is equated with freedom from the body (associated with the devalued side of the Cartesian duality). This argument extends to a desire for transgression of all 'natural' bodily boundaries. Embracing feminists' position is part of a larger pro-technology framework that transgresses limits beyond those they associate with women's non-technologically mediated reproduction. This general orientation also advocates NRTs on the basis of their ability to offer the infertile, gays/ lesbians, transsexuals/transgendereds, and persons with disabilities opportunities to overcome the limits of their 'natural' bodies and realize their desires for biologically related children, or to change sex/gender.

Embracing feminists believe the application of technology (including but not limited to NRTs) to the body dissolves boundaries such as those between man/ woman, culture/nature, society/biology, and human/machine. The cyborg, originally introduced by Donna Haraway to feminism is the iconic embodiment of this new situation as I discuss later. A fundamental part of the embracing argument is that what separates these normative categories is as discursively constituted as material. Since technology in the forms of reproductive technologies and cyberspace enable us to overcome the material base of social inequalities, they bring liberation. This logic is understandable given the history of women's oppression on the basis of their materially evident sex/gender differences from men.[57]

The defeminization of reproduction/birth is one outcome of the technology-mediated trans-dualism that embracing feminists herald. Unlike resistance feminists, they celebrate this potential as the demise of hierarchical gender and other binaries by the proliferation of identities beyond the boundaries of the physical body's characteristics, such as one's chromosomal and/or biological sex. Precisely because embracing feminists believe that female embodied reproduction is the root cause of women's oppression, they welcome futuristic projections of sex/gender-less reproduction by second-wave feminist guru Firestone in which

55 Basen et al., *Misconceptions*, Vol. 2.

56 Simone De Beauvoir, *The Second Sex*, trans. H.M. Parshley, New York: Vintage Books, 1989; Firestone, *The Dialectic of Sex*.

57 Asberg, 'Enter Cyborg', 7.

all, regardless of sex/gender share; or Marge Piercy's reproductive democracy in Mattapoisette, the fictional future society in *Woman on the Edge of Time*, a cornerstone feminist science fiction text.

Firestone is the most famous and one of the earliest proponents of NRT as liberation from the 'tyranny of reproduction'[58] unlike Simone de Beauvoir, whose anti-natalism foresaw no technological escape. That Firestone wrote the groundbreaking feminist manifesto, *The Dialectic of Sex: The Case for Feminist Revolution* in the 1960s before the advent of more advanced conceptive technologies, and spoke mainly of the 'old' (or contraceptive) forms of reproductive technology, highlights her foresight. Firestone rooted women's subjugation in their sex, or reproductive function and openly declared that *'[p]regnancy is barbaric'* calling for its abolition specifically through reproductive technology.[59] In addition, this oppression rooted in biological differences between men and women was the original form, providing a model for the class system.

Drawing from the anti-corporeal undercurrent in de Beauvoir's *The Second Sex*, Firestone believed NRTs would bring about the greatest sociopolitical revolution by destroying the material base of sex/gender difference in reproduction and thereby undermining its cultural significance. She advocated 'not just the elimination of male *privilege* but of the sex *distinction* itself'.[60] Her radical materialism led her to abolish the material foundations of cultural/political oppression rather than focusing on the redefinition and social reorganization of sex/gender difference, as have eco-feminists and radical feminists as well as the early liberal feminists.

Unlike resistance feminists, Firestone believes in the inherent threat of women's reproductive capacity to women's autonomy and liberation, and the inherent potential of technology to empower: 'like atomic energy, fertility control, artificial reproduction, cybernation, in themselves, are liberating – *unless* they are improperly used'.[61] This positive disposition towards technology as effecting good by default makes her the founder of the embracing feminist or 'technophilic' position.[62]

Firestone's pro-technology stance extends beyond NRTs. She advocates broader use of technology to fix environmental erosion. While resistance feminists argued that the techno fix approach conceals social, cultural, and economic dimensions of pollution for example, (including the industrial causes of those problems) Firestone would apply technology to fix damages that are an inevitable outcome of its processes. In keeping with her overall argument that people, not just women, have outgrown their biological constraints, she calls for 'the [technological]

---

58   Firestone, *The Dialectic of Sex*, 193.

59   Firestone, *The Dialectic of Sex*, 188.

60   Firestone, *The Dialectic of Sex*, 19.

61   Firestone, *The Dialectic of Sex*, 187.

62   Nancy Lublin, *Pandora's Box: Feminism Confronts Reproductive Technology*, Lanham, MD: Rowman and Littlefield Publishers, 1998.

establishment of a new equilibrium between man and the artificial environment he is creating, to replace the destroyed 'natural' balance'.[63]

Firestone's advocacy of women cutting their exclusive ties to biological reproduction is projected in Piercy's *Woman on the Edge of Time*. Of the revolutionary demands Firestone lists, the first is '*[t]he freeing of women from the tyranny of* reproduction by every means possible, and the diffusion of the child-rearing role to the society as a whole, to men and other children as well as women'.[64] In the fictional city, Mattapoisette, Piercy cuts women's exclusive biological ties to reproduction; Firestone believed socialist revolution had failed, at least in part, because of the failure to do this.[65] In Mattapoisette, children are birthed by machines, people are sexually ambiguous (as represented in the only pronoun 'per'), and all children have three 'mothers', not all female, who nurse them. Piercy captures the visitor from the past, Connie's, initial horror upon discovering a man breastfeeding. Her futuristic companion, Luciente, explains: 'It was part of women's long revolution. When we were breaking all the old hierarchies. Finally there was that one thing we had to give up too, the only power we ever had, in return for no more power for anyone. The original production: the power to give birth'.[66] Closely tied to the revolutionary demand to free women from childbirth is Firestone's call to do away with childhood and integrate children fully into society by socializing childrearing, echoed by Piercy.

Firestone's technophilic manifesto can be situated within a larger call for 'cybernetic communism'.[67] Her utopia was constituted of transnatural bodies, mediated by technologies that would take the ownership and control of production and reproduction out of private hands by divorcing work from wages and reproduction from women. Cybernation may be understood as 'the full takeover by machines of increasingly complex functions, altering man's age-old relation to work and wages'.[68] Together, cybernetics and reproductive technologies would break '[t]he tyranny of the biological family'.[69]

The dream of a feminist world is signified in embracing feminist literature by sex/gender-transforming technology, including technology that can be used in the service of sex/gender equality, however conceived. From the feeding bottle to *ex vivo* embryos, technology holds great potential for embracing feminists to blur the lines between culture/nature and related gender dualisms. In this context, NRTs inaugurate an era of the 'post-natural body', or the cyborg body and cyber feminism.

---

63 Lublin, *Pandora's Box*, 184.
64 Lublin, *Pandora's Box*, 221.
65 Piercy, *Woman on the Edge of Time*, 204.
66 Piercy, *Woman on the Edge of Time*, 105.
67 Firestone, *The Dialectic of Sex*, 222.
68 Firestone, *The Dialectic of Sex*, 184.
69 Firestone, *The Dialectic of Sex*.

Embracing feminists reject not only the female body, but also 'the body' as the pernicious and feminized half of the Cartesian dualism. Susan Stryker, a male-to-female transsexual theorist, depicts the distinctive character of the third wave as '"post-natural" body', illustrating the embracing feminist's position: 'the critical question for third wave feminism to address is how to deal with questions of embodied difference – whether that is specifically racial difference, sexual difference (including intersex conditions) or the kind of difference reproduced by transsexuals which I see as a precursor to a whole range of issues around biomedical technology and the 'post-natural' body'.[70]

Unlike resistance feminists, Stryker focuses on women's embodied differences from each other, rather than corporeal commonalities. Like embracing feminists in general, she scorns the woman-nature essentialism of resistance feminists. Unlike Greer, she argues that any position that generally rejects technoscience and resonates with conservative politics, is not feminist. For her, it is only when 'woman' is wrongly considered closer to 'nature' and 'man' closer to techno-culture that technology and patriarchy can be rendered synonymous, and provide the foundation for a wrongheaded feminist technophobia.

The image of the cyborg introduced in the feminist context by feminist theorist and philosopher of science and technology, Haraway, embodies the post-dualistic, post 'natural' body of embracing feminists. It is *the* feminist avatar for embracing feminists and inspires so-called cyber feminism. Given the dissolution of universal 'woman' and humanist 'man' in postmodern analysis, the cyborg became a metaphor for non-unified subjectivity. It blends Carolyn Merchant's two nature metaphors because it is both organism and 'machine', so explodes the binary structure on which these symbols are predicated.[71] This is the revolutionary, if abstract, principle on which cyber-feminism depends.[72]

Haraway introduced the cyborg in her pathbreaking postmodern 'A Cyborg Manifesto' first published in 1985.[73] The word conflates 'cybernetic and organism' and was coined by NASA research space scientists Manfred Clynes and Nathan Kline in 1960 in the context of the cold war 'space race'.[74] This is why Haraway

---

70   Susan Stryker, 'A Conversation with Susan Stryker', *International Feminist Journal of Politics* 5:1 (March 2003): 121.

71   Carolyn Merchant, *The Death of Nature: Women, Ecology and the Scientific Revolution*, San Francisco: Harper San Francisco, 1980.

72   For a good reading of two 'partly contradictory' tendencies in cyberfeminism, one inspired by Haraway's cyborg and the other 'more openly connected to a political movement', see Jenny Sunden, 'What Happened to Difference in Cyberspace? The (Re)turn of the She-Cyborg', *Feminist Media Studies* 1:2 (2001), 215–32.

73   Donna Haraway, 'A Cyborg Manifesto: Science, Technology, and Socialist-Feminism in the Late Twentieth-Century' in *Simians, Cyborgs, and Women: The Reinvention of Nature*, New York: Routledge, 1991.

74   Manfred E Clynes and Nathan S. Kline, 'Cyborgs in Space' in *The Cyborg Handbook*, ed. Chris Hables Gray, Heidi J. Figueroa-Sarriera and Steven Montor, New York and London: Routledge, 1995, 29–34.

calls it the 'illegitimate offspring of militarism and patriarchal capitalism', signifying its outlaw status, meaning outside the norm hence unthinkable, or 'monstrous', but also free to self-define.[75] To grasp Haraway's metaphor, one must first understand cybernetics as 'the study of the operation of control and communication systems' applied to both biological organisms and mechanical systems.[76] The cyborg image stresses the intimacy between organism and machine as an 'integrated circuit', an information network unhindered by boundaries and specifically the dualisms of Western enlightenment narratives. Haraway posits a post-human figure for feminists to embrace as a metaphor for the discursive material realities of being in a technological age. Human here is defined by a self-contained body clearly distinguishable from its context of techno-cultural fields. On the verge of postmodern epistemology's rise in feminism, she tells us the 'self-feminists must code' has changed into the cyborg, 'a kind of disassembled and reassembled personal self' not easily linked to a biological body.[77]

Taking cue from Haraway's ironic and iconic cyborg, cyberfeminism is a post-natural body approach to feminism, rooted in postmodern methods that puts boundary crossing to political use.[78] One tangible way in which the concept of cybernetics as embodied in the cyborg metaphor is taken up in feminism is through communications technologies and the internet. This widespread, literal cyborg experience underpins cyberfeminism (as a movement). Cyberfeminist theory is consciously directed to subversion of the female technophobic stereotype that resistance feminists (unwittingly) endorse. Sadie Plant and others decouple woman/nature and man/technology, exposing the historic and theoretical connections that women have to computers and communications systems. For instance, Plant uses Ada Lovelace, the first computer programmer, to illustrate that women are fully technologically capable.[79]

Similarly feminist theorists have analysed 'cyberspace', which is 'the fantasy world that lies beyond the hardware of the [computer] technology', as liberating for those whose embodied identifications present liabilities in patriarchal societies.[80] Cyberspace is seen as progressive because it enables women and 'others', such as people with disabilities, to free themselves from patriarchal space/time. In virtual reality, in theory, one can be whatever and whomever one wants. In reality, there

---

75   Haraway, 'A Cyborg Manifesto', 1991, 151.

76   'Cybernetics', *The New Lexicon Webster's Encyclopedic Dictionary of the English Language*, Canadian Edition, New York: Lexicon Publishers, 1988, 238.

77   Haraway, 'A Cyborg Manifesto', 1991, 163.

78   See Sunden, 'What happened to Difference in Cyberspace?'.

79   Sadie Plant, 'The Future Looms: Weaving Women and Cybernetics', in *Cybersexualities: A Reader on Feminist Theory, Cyborgs and Cyberspace*, ed. Jenny Wolmark, Edinburgh: Edinburgh University Press, 1999, 116.

80   Gibson's neologism to describe virtual reality in William Gibson, *Neuromancer*, New York: Ace Books, 1984; Sarah Gamble, *The Routledge Critical Dictionary of Feminism and Postfeminism*, New York: Routledge, 212.

are disparities in computer use/access that undermine the subversive potential of the internet.[81] Recent work also suggests the costs of a ubiquitous and insidious technoculture, nigh impossible to opt out of, is taking a potentially irreversible toll on its members.[82]

As Allucquere Stone says, while women may remain culturally associated with 'nature', technology has changed that concept. The new 'nature' that women may embody incorporates technology, like Haraway's cyborg. 'In techno-sociality, the social world of virtual culture, technics is nature'.[83] It is perhaps through the understanding that nature has been irreversibly changed by communication systems (there is no outside to technology) that the division between technology (in this case, the internet) and women can be permeated. Redefining 'nature' to include cybertechnology allows cyberfeminists to simultaneously employ and transgress deep-rooted cultural associations of women with nature.

Cyberfeminists like Plant argue that since technology disrupts traditional patriarchal binary codes, it is men who are being disempowered by new reproductive technologies, as well as by computer technologies. If patriarchy has depended on a gendered dualism that includes technology/biology, subversion of that dualism is liberatory. As we have seen, however, dualisms are always reconstructed. Stone claims that the struggle to reassert dualistic boundaries such as those between nature and culture, in which resistance feminists are engaged, is counterproductive. '[T]he project of reifying a "natural" state over and against a technologized "fallen" one is ... part of a binary, oppositional cognitive style that some maintain is part of our society's pervasively male epistemology'.[84] According to this logic, technologies that interrupt dualistic boundaries may be called feminist and progressive as Haraway's famous preference to be a cyborg rather than a goddess implies.[85]

For embracing feminists, who include but are not reducible to cyberfeminists, a feminist movement must also be technological. It must break apart the terms of patriarchal dualism (symbolically and materially) that have made women technophobes locked into a modern subject position. Severing close ties between

---

81   Dale Spender, 'The Position of Women in Information Technology – or Who Got there First and with What Consequences?' *Current Sociology*, 45:2 (1997): 135–47, and *Nattering on the Net: Women, Power and Cyberspace*, Australia: Pinifex Press Pty Ltd, 1995; Jessie Daniels, 'Rethinking Cyberfeminism(s): Race, Gender, and Embodiment', *WSQ: Women's Studies Quarterly* 37:1/2 (2009): 101–24; Bruce Bimber, 'Measuring the Gender Gap on the Internet', *Social Science Quarterly* 81:3 (2000): 868–76.

82   See Nicholas Carr, *The Shallows: How the Internet is Changing the Way We Read, Think and Remember*, London: Atlantic Books, 2010 and Heather Menzies, *No Time: Stress and the Crisis of Modern Life*, Vancouver, Canada: Douglas & McIntryre Ltd, 2005.

83   Rosanne Allucquere Stone, 'Will the Real Body Please Stand Up? Boundary Stories about Virtual Cultures', in *Cybersexualities: A Reader on Feminist Theory, Cyborgs and Cyberspace*, ed. Jenny Wolmark, Edinburgh: Edinburgh University Press, 1999, 92.

84   Stone, 'Will the Real Body Please Stand Up?', 85–6.

85   Haraway, 'A Cyborg Manifesto', 1991, 181.

organic bodies and subjectivities/identities is the hallmark of cybernetic feminism.[86] Women with disabilities provide valuable insights that foreclose easy assessments. Disability theorist Susan Wendell argues 'feminist theory has not taken account of a very strong reason for wanting to transcend the body. Unless we do take account of it, I suspect we may not only underestimate the subjective appeal of mind-body dualism, but also fail to offer an adequate alternate conception of the relationship of consciousness to the body'.[87] Her argument causes feminists to confront their dependence on a particular understanding of 'control' over their bodies and to consider the inseparability of a fuller conception of 'choice', and 'control' for some women. She reminds us over-emphasizing patriarchal control over the body (such as with NRTs in the resistance literature) permits feminists to ignore women with bodies that are chronically painful, otherwise unavoidably burdensome, or infertile. She revolutionizes traditional feminist theory of the body by forcing us to recognize that bodies are never fully under control (our own or anyone else's); will inevitably 'fail' us (we will die); and that women's bodies differ dramatically in ways that shatter normative assumptions at the foundation of feminist thought including fertility and heterosexuality as starting points in feminist resistance to NRTs.[88]

With roots in Firestone and the postmodern embrace of NRTs for their body-transcending potential, some embracing feminists argue for the use of NRTs to help people have babies that they otherwise could not, such as lesbians or gay men, men or women who are infertile and wish to be biological parents, and people with congenital disabilities (or carriers of genes for the same) which they wish to prevent passing on to their offspring. For them, reproductive 'control' requires using technology. There is a sense that the 'choice' to use NRTs should be theirs, not precluded by those (feminists included) who disapprove.[89]

For many women with disabilities, true reproductive choice is synonymous with control over their reproductive bodies given a history of eugenics, forced sterilization, de-sexualization, and other forms of denial of their sexual and reproductive agency.[90] As Gwyneth Matthews writes: 'The paradox of disabled women and sexuality goes far beyond the sexual act itself. Reproductive rights

---

86   Plant, 'The Future Looms', 116.

87   Susan Wendell. 'Feminism, Disability and Transcendence of the Body', *Canadian Woman Studies* 13:4 (Summer 1993): 118.

88   See Petra Nordqvist, 'Feminist Heterosexual Imaginaries of Reproduction: Lesbian Conception in Feminist Studies of Reproductive Technologies', *Feminist Theory* 9:3 (2008): 273–92.

89   Francie Hornstein, 'Children by Donor Insemination: A New Choice for Lesbians', in *Test-Tube Women: What Future for Motherhood.*, ed. Rita Arditti, Renate Duelli Klein and Shelley Minden, London: Pandora Press, 1989, 373. See also Nordqvist, 'Feminist Heterosexual Imaginaries of Reproduction'.

90   A. Finger, 'Claiming all of our Bodies: Reproductive Rights and Disability', in *Test-Tube Women*, ed. Arditti, Klein and Minden; D. Kaplan, 'Disability Rights Perspectives on Reproductive Technologies and Public Policy', in *Reproductive Laws for the 1990s*, ed. Nadine Taub and Sherrill Cohen, New Brunswick: Rutgers University, 1988, 241–7.

... [for them] ... include the right to have a baby, the right to adopt children, the right not to have children and to have access to abortion clinics' among others.[91] Matthews interviewed 45 women with disabilities for *Voices from the Shadows*. In a chapter called 'Bringing up Baby', it is clear that many women interviewed would consider abortion if prenatal diagnosis revealed a congenital defect: 'I asked some of the younger women who might possibly face [the dilemma of discovering a genetic defect *in utero*]. Not one said she would *never* consider abortion, but most admitted to mixed feelings. ... they wouldn't mind having disabled children, but they would be terrified for the children's sake'.[92] Similarly, Virginia Kallianes and Phyllis Rubenfeld note the counter-intuitive results of a survey on selective abortion: 'a survey on attitudes toward abortion among mothers of congenitally disabled children and mothers of non-disabled children found very similar responses: while some of the mothers of disabled children opposed selective abortions, both groups of mothers also supported abortion at similar rates'.[93] These embracing feminist positions reveal the difficult ethical dimensions of 'freedom of choice' and its centrality for women's reproductive autonomy.

Since embracing feminists consider choice an inextricable part of women's reproductive control, it is impossible to limit women's technological options within their framework. Even the more pragmatic arguments are based on those of Firestone and de Beauvoir, which see the body as oppressive and seek to transcend it. Can embracing feminism transform that approach's body-phobic inheritance, plus postmodern anti-essentialism, into a more reproduction-affirming feminist currency? Perhaps the question should be posed in terms of its ability to address patriarchal economies in which techno-embracing currencies will inevitably be circulated. There are good reasons to be concerned that despite embracing feminists' attempted dissolution of the patriarchal categories that make women technophobes and men technomanics, in strongly advocating technology such as NRTs and cyberspace they end up reinforcing what they intend to undo. They run the risk of reasserting patriarchal dualism in the form of technology over 'nature' which retains an essentialist significance in spite of its thorough renunciation and reconceptualization in feminist cultures. Most importantly, what does this technological embrace contribute to a birth-appropriative history in the West that encourages women to transcend their bodies in exchange for citizenship and power?

---

91   Gwyneth F. Matthews, *Voices From the Shadows: Women with Disabilities Speak Out*, Toronto: The Women's Press, 1983, 16.

92   Matthews, *Voices from the Shadows*, 102.

93   Virginia Kallianes and Phyllis Rubenfeld, 'Disabled Women and Reproductive Rights', *Disability & Society* 12:2 (1997): 213. See also Rayna Rapp's account of her own experience aborting a second trimester, genetically diagnosed foetus in 'XYLO: A True Story' in *Test-Tube Women*, ed. Arditti, Klein and Minden, 326.

Conclusion – Choice, Control and/or Reproductive Justice?

There are two prominent and apparently opposed feminist discourses that have emerged in response to NRTs, and a third which mediates them in many respects as I will examine in the following chapter. Each has a different notion of liberation shaped by the patriarchal logic of value dualism (especially man/technology over woman/nature), and is further circumscribed by 'choice' and 'control' over the body rooted in feminist Anglo-American politics. The theory and practice of feminists who resist and embrace NRTs are therefore easily evaluated on the basis of their abilities to transcend patriarchal dualism; this includes tensions between women's common and diverse experiences of reproduction. In a broader conceptual framework these are associated with essentialism and anti-essentialism respectively.

Both embracing feminists and resistance feminists reasserted patriarchal dualism and fostered an essentialized notion of 'woman' associated with 'nature' on the basis of her reproductive functions. In other respects these two positions are quite distinct. Resisters celebrate women's reproduction and oppose technologies as patriarchal tools usurping women's control over their own bodies. For them, protecting women's reproductive control and autonomy, collectively, justifies subordination of the rights of individual women and their choices to use NRTs. Resistance feminists perceive control and choice oppositionally, arguing for women's 'right to control [their] bodies and reproduction rather than freedom of individual choice'.[94] They comment on the power of the 'choice' discourse to discipline feminist opinion by positioning anyone who opposes NRTs as 'against a woman's right to choose'.[95] Resisters are particularly vociferous in arguing that 'choice' is socially constructed and that 'the new reproductive technologies actually restrict the range of choices available to women with disabilities specifically and non-disabled women generally'.[96] This is so, they argue, because NRTs ultimately reinforce normative understandings of who should reproduce and what sorts of offspring they should have; NRTs which aid in the production of able-bodied and 'perfect' children are to be encouraged while others are to be discouraged.

The embracers, rooted in Firestone's bio-phobic embrace of reproductive technology, welcome NRTs to help women overcome the limits of their natural bodies, thereby granting them control through greater choice. Embracers conflate control and choice, meaning that women's control over their reproductive bodies requires choice, including the choice *to bear children*. This issue is more significant to women with disabilities, lesbians, and infertile women who, without NRTs, may be unable to bear children and/or have less control over the variables affecting their decisions. For example, although the most visible position on NRTs

---

94 Judy Rebick, 'Is the Issue Choice?', in Basen et al., *Misconceptions*, Vol. 1, p. 89.
95 Basen et al., *Misconceptions*, Vol. 1, p. 169; See also Louise Vandelac, 'The Industrialization of Life', in Basen et al., *Misconceptions*, Vol. 2.
96 Vandelac, in Basen et al., *Misconceptions*, Vol. 2, p. 154.

by persons with disabilities is characterized by concerns about their eugenic potential, many women at higher risk of conceiving children with disabilities welcome prenatal diagnostic technologies that allow them to choose whether or not to birth such a child, or to better prepare for its arrival. Ultimately, 'control', for feminists who embrace NRTs, requires women's ability to use technology to meet their reproductive needs.

The simultaneous feminist resistance to NRTs and acceptance of old reproductive technologies by some feminists highlights how 'choice' is a problematic strategic discourse from the point of view of contemporary reproductive politics and in an important allegorical way clarifies and magnifies the tension between the embrace of, and resistance to, NRTs. Even within the earlier context of abortion politics in North America, the language was fraught with difficulty indicating a deeper problem with its feminist appropriation. The language of 'choice' presents a number of difficulties related to its invocation of a market logic that individualizes reproductive rights that ought to be guaranteed collectively. Choice is not the same as rights as is highlighted by abortion funding in the US: 'abortion was framed as a consumer service that the government could not prevent a woman from getting but one that it also would not help to fund. Thus abortion became a consumer choice but not a guaranteed right for all women'.[97] In this context 'choice' has been shown to undermine feminism because it reduces significantly complex differences between women to polar and antagonistic subject positions. For example, the language of choice has been used to distinguish between '"legitimate choice-making mothers" (for example, with post-secondary education, financial stability and in heterosexual relationships) and "bad choice-making mothers" (for example, socio-economically disadvantaged, single or of uncertain relationship status and orientation)'.[98]

Furthermore, it individualizes maternal politics, and their consequences, by using the language of the free market with the underlying assumption that all have equal access to the benefits of (and the ability to minimize burdens related to) reproduction, as well as the resources needed to reproduce in the first place. In this way it conceals the systemic bias that gives certain women access to legitimate motherhood while excluding others.

Mainstream reproductive discourse, and feminist theories of reproduction that offer women better lives via 'control' over their reproductive bodies, beg the question: what notion of liberation underlies 'better lives' based on NRTs? I agree with the resisting feminists that the association of power with control (over nature) is too steeped in scientific models historically abusive to women, to be uncritically adopted by feminists. The very question of 'control' over women's reproduction, not to mention who will get to have it and when, depends upon a specific conceptualization of the problem of women's subordination as rooted in

---

97   Mary Thompson, 'Third Wave Feminism and the Politics of Motherhood', *Genders OnLine Journal* 43 (2006): 10.

98   Thompson, 'Third Wave Feminism', 1.

their reproductive bodies and consciousnesses. It also exposes a partial perspective that may distort issues of embodiment which are of fundamental importance to feminism. Wendell (1988) reminds us that bodies are not only sources of pleasure to be simply 'reclaimed' for women, and debunks the myth of western medicine that we *can* 'control' our bodies.

Aware of the pitfalls of both choice and control discourse when applied to NRTs, how can we transcend that paradigm for reproductive justice more attuned to the differences amongst women, including between those who use the technology and those who do not? The experience of lesbians building families with these technologies can be instructive here as Yeung writes: 'reproductive justice is a more useful frame when discussing [technology and policy] than the choice frame. ... [because it], allows us to focus on something we haven't, which is the connection to supporting women to have kids, not just choose not to have kids'.[99] This is a helpful counter to the anti-natalist thread of some 'second wave' feminism, including but not limited to Beauvoir and Firestone.

En route to a theory of reproductive justice, a robust material feminism would build on the equivocal position that finds a mean between the extremes of resistance to, and full embrace of, NRTs. This material feminist account of NRTs enables an incorporation of the diversity of women's individual reproductive experiences (because it starts from it), while still accounting for the corporeal commonalities women share.

Ultimately, any kind of argument for a viable reproductive justice must recognize the bio-social character of reproduction of such thinkers as O'Brien, Carol Stabile and Nancy Lublin. It is to these that we turn next in the equivocal feminist response to NRTs.

---

99   Miriam Yeung, 'Conceiving the Future: Reproductive-justice Activists on Technology and Policy', *Bitch: Feminist Response to Pop Culture* 40 (2008): 58–63.

Chapter 3
Equivocals

The equivocal feminist response to new reproductive technologies (NRTs) serves as both a deep critique and negotiation of the feminists who resist and those who embrace the NRTs as discussed in the previous chapter. Equivocal feminists assert that while women have been subjugated collectively on the basis of bodily reproductive functions, they are differently affected according to their specific locations in ethnic, socio-economic, and other communities. They develop a middle ground position regarding female reproduction and mothering, and technology and NRTs, arguing that the latter are neither inherently oppressive nor liberating. Taking a practical approach to the NRTs, they recognize the reality of their widespread use and seek to regulate them in support of a broad range of women's reproductive needs.

Equivocal feminists assess the two responses to NRTs discussed in the previous chapter as partial because of their polarized character.[1] This critique is implicit in the neologisms that Carol Stabile uses to describe resistance and embracing feminist positions, as 'technophobia' and 'technomania' (or 'technophilia') respectively.[2] Adding the implications for feminist agency of both positions in terms of women's control, Heather Menzies offers 'an attempt to break the dichotomy which positions us either outside the technology with no opportunity to control it, or totally within its control, little more than helpless victims'.[3] Biologic and dualistic accounts of both technophobes and technophiles ultimately conflate woman/nature by rooting women's relationship to technology (NRT) in a flight from, or wholesale embrace of, their 'natural' bodies. By contrast, equivocal feminists promote a biosocial understanding of reproduction and mothering, and a feminist strategy incorporating the diversity of women's experiences to bridge theory and practice.[4] The common element is a requirement that feminist responses be rooted in the actual circumstances of women's reproductive lives as inscribed by social and material structures of constraint if also of agency. Consequently,

---

1   Michelle Stanworth, ed., *Reproductive Technologies: Gender, Motherhood and Medicine*, Minneapolis: University of Minnesota Press, 1987, 3.

2   See Nancy Lublin, *Pandora's Box: Feminism Confronts Reproductive Technology*, Lanham, MD: Rowman and Littlefield Publishers, 1998.

3   Gwynne Basen, Margrit Eichler and Abby Lippman, eds, *Misconceptions: The Social Construction of Choice and the New Reproductive and Genetic Technologies*, Vol. 1, Prescott, Ontario: Voyageur Publishing, 1993.

4   Carol Stabile, *Feminism and the Technological Fix*, Manchester: Manchester University Press, 1994; Lublin, *Pandora's Box*.

equivocalists often develop a materialist feminist account of NRTs, indebted to Marxist/socialist principles to incorporate the diversity of women's individual reproductive experiences, while capturing the corporeal commonalities women share. As such, at the conceptual level there is something deeper, and promisingly trans-dualistic at play that has to do with the renaissance of materialism in the new material feminisms, to which I will return in Part III.

Claiming that technophobia's essentialism and technomania's anti-essentialism only misleadingly suggest 'distinct trajectories', Stabile argues that in reality, 'technophobia and technomania illustrate the continuing dualism at the heart of contemporary feminist thought: an ideology based on gender differences versus an ideology based on the endless and multiple play of difference'.[5] Feminist responses conform to patriarchal dualities that either embrace technologies as good, and conceive of women as not essentially the same despite their shared corporeality ('technomanics'), or reject technologies as bad for women as a cohesive and homogenous group based on their shared corporeality ('technophobes'). Before the *Cyborg Manifesto*, Haraway's earlier work, *Situated Knowledges: The Science Question in Feminism and the Privilege of Partial Perspective*, reinforced the equivocals' argument here. Making her case for situated knowledges that are constituted of consciously employed partial perspectives in feminism, she positions them as the mediation of relativism and universalism, corollaries of the dualism we are concerned with as underpinning the resistance and embracing responses. Though she applied her analysis to scientific epistemology (most directly) she speaks of the same dualistic dynamic I do when she writes, 'Relativism is the perfect mirror twin of totalization in the ideologies of objectivity; *both deny the stakes in location, embodiment, and partial perspective*; both make it impossible to see well'.[6]

Building on Stabile's argument, Nancy Lublin critiques the 'basic assumption' of the technomanic position as the over-privileging of sexual dualism as the primary, most significant source of women's oppression, especially as represented by Shulamith Firestone. She asserts that Firestone's resultant biophobic prescription for doing away with biological/sexual difference to achieve equality between the sexes is 'an overly simplistic approach to such pervasive inequality' but it has bequeathed its biases to the technomanic branch of feminism.[7] Despite the prominence of the cyborg metaphor in postmodern feminist theory, it is 'a cyborg ... that, in what might be construed as the apex of anti-essentialist thought,

---

5   Stabile, *Feminism and the Technological Fix*, 44.

6   Donna Haraway, 'Situated Knowledges: The Science Question in Feminism and the Privilege of Partial Perspective', *Feminist Studies* 14:3 (1988): 575–99. Emphasis added.

7   Lublin, *Pandora's Box*, 35–6. For a more recent and alternative reading of Shulamith Firestone's legacy see Mandy Merck and Stella Sandford, *Further Adventures of The Dialectic of Sex: Critical Essays on Shulamith Firestone*, Basingstoke: Palgrave Macmillan, 2010.

threatens completely to overwhelm material female bodies'.[8] Equivocal feminists like Stabile are among the many feminists dubious about the cyborg's playful, theoretical boundary-crossing as a method to adequately address the material issues presented to women in the era of new reproductive technology.

Equivocal feminists are as critical of the technophobic position as they are of the technomanic. Lublin, Stabile, and others critique the association of an ideological conception of 'woman' with an equally mystified notion of 'nature' most clearly exemplified in eco-feminist theory. 'When technology stands in opposition to women (who by virtue of their anatomical configuration have special links with nature), technology functions like the term patriarchy' with its universalizing and (biological) determinist undertones.[9] But the dualism technophobia maintains dissolves in the face of often contradictory and intersecting historical and material realities.[10] Because biology's deterministic connotations are so deeply embedded in western culture, its unqualified invocation perpetuates rather than mitigates false and gendered dualism. In fact, however, corporeality (the experience of embodied life) is connected across such tensions, as is best illustrated in Shiloh Whitney's analysis of the vulnerability – power duality in reference to both feminist and orthodox political thought, something that I return to in the conclusion.

The equivocal position, then, overlaps with aspects of the positions of both embracers and resisters. For example, like resisters, equivocalists critique the 'techno fix' approach for downplaying the socio-economic contexts and causes of problems NRTs are supposed to remedy. A science-and-techno-centric focus of NRT discourses detracts from the greater social dilemmas and frameworks that present obstacles to women's reproductive autonomy including but not limited to 'the legal system which frames our rights over our bodies and our children, from political struggles over the nature of sexuality, parenthood and the family and from the impact of the varied material and cultural circumstances in which people create their personal lives'.[11] By contrast, equivocal feminists call on women to confront the material conditions of their embodied lives, which are only partially defined by their sex/gender. For example, Rosalind Petchesky notes that '[t]he majority of poor and working-class women in the United States and Britain still have no access to amniocentesis, IVF and the rest, although they (particularly women of colour) have the highest rates of infertility and foetal impairment'.[12] 'Technophiles' celebrate the multiple sites of identification of the postmodern subject, and to a great extent, this is what allows women to interface anew with the technologies, yet the ideological/textual nature of their theory circumscribes their ability to speak to the diverse material conditions of women's lives. While many

---

8   Stabile, *Feminism and the Technological Fix*, 93.
9   Stabile, *Feminism and the Technological Fix*, 52.
10   Stabile, *Feminism and the Technological Fix*, 52.
11   Stabile, *Feminism and the Technological Fix*, 4.
12   Cited in Stabile, *Feminism and the Technological Fix*, 77.

women embrace technology, such as NRTs, socio-economic and other conditions that shape this relationship are inadequately assessed in a 'techno fix' approach.

Equivocal feminists investigate reproductive technology with an emphasis on the present material conditions of reproduction and existing technologies which further dispels any erroneous belief in the uniformity of women's experiences of NRTs whether perceived as positive or negative. Although much theory and talk about reproductive technology inspires science fiction narrative, Hilary Rose asks feminists to take a cool-headed approach to the fantasy elements of NRTs.[13] Unlike 'techno-determinists', she thinks it is important for feminists to concern themselves with the technologies that are part of women's lives and those likely to be developed, rather than ascribing more power to technology than it has.[14] For example, genetic screening and gene therapy are greater and more immediate concerns for women than future prospects like ectogenesis, cloning, and male maternity, which capture a disproportionate amount of attention in popular and political discourse.[15]

Since, for equivocal feminists 'blanket acceptance or rejection is no substitute for informed and critical appraisal', each technology must be assessed for its merit, accounting for multiple reproductive experiences.[16] Starting from the irreducibly complex relationship women have to their bodies and technology, there is no single theoretical framework that can account for and regulate all women's relationships to NRT all of the time.[17] First and foremost, equivocal feminists argue that women must engage with techno-science, and its difficult debates, and not avoid them out of hand.[18] In contrast to 'technophobes', for example, they legitimize the voices and concerns of infertile women whose choices and opinions, they believe, are irreducible to the symptoms of social inequalities (as resistance feminists would have it). Petchesky asks: 'Are lesbians [or women with disabilities?] to be told that wanting their "own biological children" generated through their own bodies is somehow wrong for them but not for fertile heterosexual couples?'[19] In the journal *Trouble and Strife* Naomi Pfeffer responded to FINRRAGE's (Feminist International Network of Resistance to Reproductive and Genetic Engineering)

---

13   Cited in Stabile, *Feminism and the Technological Fix.*

14   Cited in Stabile, *Feminism and the Technological Fix*, 159.

15   See Candace Johnson, 'The Political 'Nature' of Pregnancy and Childbirth', *The Canadian Journal of Political Science* 41:4 (December 2008) for a discussion of the class and psychological aspects of calls for 'natural' childbirth.

16   Johnson, 'The Political 'Nature of Pregnancy and Childbirth', 3.

17   Johnson, 'The Political Nature of Pregnancy and Childbirth', 35.

18   Stanworth, 'Reproductive Technologies and the Deconstruction of Motherhood' and Rose, 'Victorian Values in the Test-Tube: The Politics of Reproductive Science and Technology', in Stanworth, *Reproductive Technologies.*

19   Petchesky, 'Foetal Images: The Power of Visual Culture in the Politics of Reproduction', in Stanworth, *Reproductive Technologies.* See also Petra Nordqvist, 'Feminist Heterosexual Imaginaries of Reproduction: Lesbian Conception in Feminist Studies of Reproductive Technologies', *Feminist Theory* 9:3 (2008).

proposal for a moratorium on NRTs objecting to what she called, 'the advocacy of totalitarian policies because they are based on theory, rather than real experience'.[20] Furthermore, she rejected the characterization of infertile women as weak, 'desperate, coerced, or prey to false consciousness'.[21] The false notion of the 'natural' (including heterosexual and fertile) woman at the foundation of the technophobic position dismisses women who want to use technology.[22]

The Canadian Royal Commission on New Reproductive Technologies

Eschewing moratoriums and the lack of regulation of NRTs equally, the equivocalists need a way to evaluate the possible harms and/or benefits a given technology poses for women and their families. Lublin provides a good summary: 'Although a comprehensive feminist framework is needed, it should be a set of standards against which particular technologies can be measured'.[23] Eichler provides such as the leader of the group lobbying for a Canadian Coalition for a Royal Commission in the spring of 1987, providing criteria as regulatory guidelines for NRTs in the absence of federal legislation.[24] The eight principles reflect an equivocal feminist, middle-ground position between absolute rejection and unconditional acceptance of NRTs. The first item is quintessential: '*Each reproductive technology needs to be evaluated separately with respect to its overall social desirability*'.[25] Eichler provides the example of sex-preselection techniques, arguing that contrary to popular opinion, there are situations in which such procedures would be 'desirable' such as 'if the gametes of a couple carried a genetic illness that appears in one sex but not in the other'.[26]

Since Eichler's article was published, the Royal Commission on NRTs (RCNRTs) was established, in 1989. After considerable conflict and controversy it published a lengthy report called *Proceed with Care* in 1993, which contains elements of an equivocal position on NRTs in that it officially gives voice to more than one position. The intense controversy surrounding the commission's administration, methodology, and leadership, however, renders suspect its putative

---

20   Naomi Pfeffer, 'Not so New Technologies', *Trouble and Strife* 5 (1985): 46–50. See also Pfeffer, *The Stork and the Syringe: A Political History of Reproductive Medicine*, Cambridge: Polity Press, 1993; and cited in Lublin, *Pandora's Box*, 68.

21   Cited in Pfeffer, 'Not so New Technologies', 68. See also Marge Berer who agreed with Pfeffer in the same publication.

22   See Nordqvist, 'Feminist Heterosexual Imaginaries of Reproduction', 273–92.

23   Nordqvist, 'Feminist Heterosexual Imaginaries of Reproduction'.

24   Christine Overall, ed., *The Future of Human Reproduction*, Toronto: The Women's Press, 1989, 226.

25   Overall, *The Future of Human Reproduction*.

26   Overall, *The Future of Human Reproduction*.

feminist and egalitarian character.[27] Conflicts between some commissioners and the chair led to the unprecedented firing of four commissioners; the commission's recommendations and practices were subsequently rejected and criticized by prominent feminist and social science organizations, including the National Action Committee on the Status of Women (NAC), and the Social Science Federation of Canada (SSFC). Assessments about the nature of the conflict vary, but most focus on how the chair, Dr Patricia Baird (a physician), conducted the research and administration. Many feminists argue that Baird's 'autocratic' research and management style, and her expertise in genetic epidemiology, resulted in privileging the techno-medical and commercial interest to the detriment of all others.[28] Some members of the research staff 'focused on personality conflicts among Commissioners arising from the political process of choosing the Chairperson'.[29] Others criticized the report's liberal framework and rhetorical appropriation of feminist terms. Annette Burfoot, for example, criticized the report for appropriating feminist 'concerns' while denying 'their political origins'.[30] She observes that '[t]he only political approach evident in the Report is liberal, especially in regard to choice'.[31] Likely the truth is a combination of varying perspectives. Despite its difficult origins, the appropriately titled *Proceed with Care* reflects an equivocal position on NRTs and provides an official framework by which to evaluate each technology on the basis of its individual and social consequences, albeit through a lens not unequivocally or unambiguously feminist.

Although indisputably problematic, the commission laid the groundwork for public discourse and policy that incorporates a framework in keeping with equivocal feminism. This is clear in its discourse, recommendations, and the legislation based on them. For example, the inquiry adopted an 'ethic of care' approach (as opposed to implicit liberal individualism) and treated technologies separately to attempt to 'balanc[e] individual and collective interests'.[32] Its recommendations attempt to prevent commodification of reproduction, especially

---

27   For more on the controversy, see Maureen McTeer, *In My Own Name: A Memoir*, Canada: Random House, 2003; Basen et al., *Misconceptions*, 1993; Annette Burfoot, 'In-Appropriation – A Critique of "Proceed With Care: Final Report of the Royal Commission on New Reproductive Technologies"', *Women's Studies International Forum* 18:4 (1995): 499–506.; Mariana Valverde and Lorna Weir, 'Regulating New Reproductive and Genetic Technologies: A Feminist View of Recent Canadian Government Initiatives', *Feminist Studies* 23:2 (1997); and Francesca Scala, 'Experts, Non-Experts and Policy Discourse: A Case Study of the Royal Commission on New Reproductive Technologies' (Ph.D. Diss.), Carleton University, Ottawa, 2002.

28   Mariana Valverde and Lorna Weir, 'Regulating New Reproductive and Genetic Technologies'.

29   Scala, *Experts, Non-Experts and Policy Discourse*, 167.

30   Burfoot, 'In-Appropriation', 500.

31   Burfoot, 'In-Appropriation', 501.

32   Patricia Baird, 'New Reproductive Technologies: The Canadian Perspective', *Women's Health Issues* 6:3 (1996): 158.

pertinent for women, as individuals and as a class, and something demanded by feminists who lobbied the commission.

The commission conducted its inquiry from the starting point that 'reproductive technologies are not a monolith'.[33] Its 'ethic of care' approach arguably influenced the new policy however dissociated from its feminist base. Baird explains the methodology as 'a stance that gives priority to the mutual care and connectedness between people and their communities'.[34] More practically, the commission's report concluded that some techniques needed to be banned and others regulated since '[i]ndividual decisions regarding use of reproductive technology (such as in vitro fertilization or prenatal diagnosis) may be personally beneficial, yet have undesirable collective consequences'.[35] Perhaps the most important recommendation of the commission was for the establishment of an independent regulatory body. Furthermore, the commission's recommendations to ban technologies such as cloning and ectogenesis, while allowing the regulated use of in vitro fertilization and sex-selection (only for sex-linked genetic diseases) are justified by the mandate to 'balanc[e] individual and collective interests'. This justification is significant for my analysis when interpreted as individual women's needs versus women-as-a-group's needs. Though the criteria by which a technology may be deemed beneficial or harmful for an individual or community may not be universally agreed upon, the commission's recommendations attempt to address the concerns of most Canadians, and if not the majority of feminists at least those holding an equivocal position. In 2004, the Canadian *Act Respecting Assisted Human Reproduction and Related Research* (AHRA) was passed, and implemented all major recommendations of the Royal Commission on NRTs.

For equivocal feminists, women's control of their reproduction involves the ability to choose, within reason, how to govern it; this includes using technologies that provide options for individual women and are not harmful to the social whole. It also involves regulating NRTs which could be dangerous and banning others outright. At the same time, equivocal feminists recognize the socio-economic and political dimensions of NRTs and call for social transformations of inequitable circumstances that mean that not all women experience the technology as beneficial. What distinguishes the equivocal attempts at regulation from the position of resistance feminists is that they allow for the assessment of technologies individually, rather than calling for complete moratoriums as demanded by FINRRAGE and NAC.[36] The commission's recommendations, which were subsequently enshrined in Canadian law are an equivocal feminist position on NRTs in that they eschew either a wholesale embrace of or resistance to technologies and promote an approach that both prohibits and regulates certain

---

33 Baird, 'New Reproductive Technologies', 163.

34 Baird, 'New Reproductive Technologies', 158.

35 Baird, 'New Reproductive Technologies', 156.

36 Both of these organizations presented briefs to the RCNRTs to this effect. See Basen et al., *Misconceptions*.

technologies based on a liberal reading of an ethics of care. In addition to this liberal position vis-à-vis policy creation, the equivocalist's theoretical heritage is more heterogeneous as we will see next.

Theoretical Foundations

The equivocals offer a feminist response to NRTs traceable to Marxist/socialist principles, especially class analysis (traditionally economic class, but later including sex class) and historical (or dialectical) materialism – as a methodology and worldview. While a full account of Marxism and the evolution of socialist feminism out of Marxist principles is impossible here, to understand the equivocal position (and the new material feminisms with which they overlap) we must undertake a selective explanation. Marx believed that lived material realities have a formative role in the way we think. His materialism is the idea that the nature of relations between people in society is a function of its economy or the way we reproduce our social and material existence every day. He believed that it is not what we think that determines what we do, but what we do that determines what and how we think.[37]

Michelle Stanworth and others like her exhibit these socialist principles in making central the social, political and economic contexts of NRT's development and use, and so of women's experiences of them. The priority is the ways in which our experiences are shaped not simply by desires and beliefs but also material structures (like policies that would prohibit single women and lesbians from using IVF, or the high costs associated with them.) For Marxists, historical materialism accords 'material forces – the production and reproduction of social life' the central role in historical process, change and society. Of course these structures variously affect women according to their different, usually complex and overlapping, social locations; in a phrase their class memberships including, but not limited to, socio-economic class in the traditional Marxist sense.

Socialist feminism evolved from Marxist feminism and has affinities with radical feminism. As such it maintains a historic tension between its constituent components of Marxism's focus on capitalism and radical feminism's focus on patriarchy as the sources of women's oppression in modern life.[38] This history is important: socialist feminists insist on the interrelated oppressions of capitalism

---

37   Marx wrote: 'The mode of production of material life conditions the social, political and intellectual life process in general. It is not the consciousness of men that determines their being, but, on the contrary, their social being that determines their consciousness', Karl Marx and Friedrich Engels, 'Preface to the Critique of Political Economy'. *Selected Works*, London: Lawrence and Wishart, 1968, 182.

38   For more, see Rosemarie Tong, *Feminist Thought: A More Comprehensive Introduction*, Boulder, CO: Westview Press, 1998; Marysia Zalewski, *Feminism after Postmodernism: Theorising through Practice*, London and New York: Routledge, 2000;

and patriarchy rather than analytically privileging one or the other. Individuals' actions are taken as embedded in combined sociopolitical, historical, and economic contexts, themselves characterized by patriarchal capitalist forces. For socialist feminists the institutions of science and medicine, and the (new reproductive) technologies produced by them, are similarly structured by these forces (if not determined by them.)

Over time and specifically with the publication of Juliet Mitchell's *Women: The Longest Revolution* (1966), as well as the famous insights of Carol Gilligan (1982) and Nancy Chodorow (1978), socialist feminism incorporated a psychoanalytic component to its materialist analysis. The way the world's structures and institutions circumscribed women's experiences were, then, not so easily distinguished from ideological and psychological constructs. This interrelation is a hallmark of post-structural theory or postmodernism as I refer to it here. In fact, and in spite of the supposed 'theoretical gulf' between postmodernist and modernist impulses in feminism, Zalewski writes, '[postmodernism's] emphasis on the constructive nature of meaning and reality arguably links it with the historical materialist approaches of socialist feminism'.[39] Both focus on the process of experiencing the world as in structures versus agency, but differently characterize that process with postmodern's privileging discourse, and Marxist socio-economic and socio-cultural structures. This is a crucial point in my argument that has to do with the ideological roots of the new material feminisms so warrants fuller treatment in the next two chapters.

Socialist feminism's 'special contribution' of feminist standpoint theory, developed by scholars like Nancy Hartsock (1983), Dorothy Smith (1987) and Sandra Harding (1986, 1987, 1991) was one result of its foray into psychoanalytic theory.[40] Feminist standpoint theory, also known as feminist standpoint epistemology, is materialist in a Marxist sense because it is based on the idea that what we do shapes who we are (rather than the other way around). It is based in the understanding that all knowledge is partial since it is constituted of life experiences which differ, and that sex/gender shapes women's and men's experiences as distinct. In addition, the epistemological position of the feminist subject gives her an epistemically privileged knowledge, compared to men's

and Gillian Howies, *Between Feminism and Materialism: A Question of Method*, New York: Palgrave Macmillan, 2010.

39   Zalewski, *Feminism after Postmodernism*, 133. See also Iris van der Tuin, 'Deflationary Logic: Response to Sara Ahmed's "Imaginary Prohibitions: Some Preliminary Remarks on the Founding Gestures of the 'New Materialism'"', *European Journal of Women's Studies* 15:4 (2008) 411–16.

40   There is continuity between post-structuralism and standpointism which is manifest in the new material feminisms. But this is no singular, linear or teleological linkage and subverts such characterization. Ultimately this exercise of assigning theoretical pedigree to standpointism is important insofar as its heterogeneity serves to unify/point out the common ground of many otherwise diverse (even antagonistic) theoretical traditions. See Van der Tuin, 'Deflationary Logic', 414–15.

because, in theory, it is a historically subjugated way of seeing less invested in upholding the patriarchal status quo.[41] It should be noted that feminist standpoint has a long history in Western feminist theory and has been well-debated as to whether it can be attributed to women, simply by virtue of her experiences of such a gendered embodiment, or involves the critical reflection on those experiences. I defer to Hartsock's original concept, who clarifies it involves analysis, so is an achievement that is 'struggled for' rather than simply an unreflective point of view. Furthermore, and significantly – the standpoint of the disadvantaged or the 'view from below' implies a recognition that there are multiple views (since one recognizes one's standpoint as a misfit between dominant narratives and one's personal experience of the world) hence is already counter-hegemonic in the sense of challenging the single-track, God's eye view underpinning much of modern normative thought.

Feminist standpoint is a complex theory that examines the many ways in which women's lives differ from men's, but women's experience of the separation of public and private spheres runs through most of the points of distinction. Feminist standpoint theorists took Marx's materialist insight that 'we are what we do' to argue that women's daily immersion in the necessities of existence (the washing, cooking, childcare and such) gives them a unique perspective on the world, unavailable to most men and one that is necessary, if not sufficient, for progressive change;[42] something that a recent popular news article on the 'chore wars' as the 'last bastion' of male privilege (at least for upper middle class women) might support.[43] Mary O'Brien's focused work on reproduction takes this view further in replacing Marx's productive relations as the driving force of history, with reproductive relations (as I will explore). But in a sense, all feminist theories that prioritize women's perspectives, regardless of their justification for it, and whether it distinguishes women primarily from men or from other women, are making a claim on the basis of standpoint theory.

While feminist standpoint epistemology was brought to account for its potentially essentialist underpinnings in the postmodern turn, we may see its basic features re-remerging in some new feminist theories, specifically those addressing the issue of feminism's twenty-first-century relevance, as well as of embodiment and the biology/society debate that I focus on here. For example mother and daughter feminist scholars, Kath and Sophie Woodward, conclude their excellent *Why Feminism Matters* with a call for a 'reversioned standpoint epistemology which focuses on the specificities of gendered situations'.[44] In addition, socialist

---

41   Van der Tuin, 'Deflationary Logic', 51.

42   Zalewski, *Feminism after Postmodernism*, 52.

43   Tralee Pearce, 'Ending the Chore War: 5 Ideas for Peace on the Domestic Front', *The Globe and Mail*, 6 June 2013. Online.

44   Woodward and Woodward, *Why Feminism Matters*, 170. See also Rosemarie Garland-Thomson, 'Misfits: A Feminist Materialist Disability Concept', *Hypatia* 26:3 (2011); and Gillian Howie, *Between Feminism and Materialism*, 205 where each call for

feminist ideas are alive in the (new) material feminisms. For example, Gillian Howie's reconsideration of the relationship of materialism and feminism is a *tour de force*. She concludes: 'to form political alliances we need to account for located situated knowledge and to map the systematic nature of interests: we need both a respect for differences and to know which differences are relevant'.[45] These critically important theoretical advancements will be given further consideration in the next chapter.[46]

As a side note, it is worth mentioning that during the 1980s when O'Brien was writing and Somer Brodribb – Mary's student – first applied reproductive consciousness to NRT, there was a key split among feminists, especially in the UK regarding IVF (and related technologies). It is typically described as radical feminists, or resistors in my framing (including for example Gena Corea, and Patricia Spallone) versus socialist feminists, or equivocals (like Michelle Stanworth and Lynda Birke). Although this argument predates the term, the radical feminist faction, which ironically included O'Brien who is recognized as a socialist feminist, was subsequently charged with essentialism. These tensions indicate clashing interpretations, and placements of various arguments indicates the complicated intersectionality and heritage of feminist positions on NRT – and reinforce a hermeneutic reading of feminist texts and arguments. Annette Burfoot adds a more prosaic dimension in suggesting limited funding opportunities and publication routes, and varying levels of success in attaining them between these two feminist approaches may have also played a part in the dispute.[47] Nonetheless, such contestations within feminism, highlight the conceptual differences and overlaps that are explicitly addressed in the present material turn as I explore in Chapter 5.

Conclusion

The socialist/materialist approach goes by many names in the equivocal feminist response to NRTs; important here are Lublin's 'praxis feminism',[48] 'materialist

---

a version of standpoint feminism via a self-consciously situated theory. See, Haraway in 'Situated Knowledges' where she calls for a feminist objectivity that recognizes partial perspective.

45   Howie, *Between Feminism and Materialism*, 204.

46   I want to emphasize that I use 'advancements' in a qualified sense here because the exciting developments the new material feminisms represent also draw on the history of feminist thought (for example Harding and Haraway) in a way that breaks apart the linear and teleological sense of the term.

47   Annette Burfoot, 'Feminist Technoscience: A Solution to Theoretic Conundrums and the Wane of Feminist Politics?', *Resources for Feminist Research*, 33:3 (2010): 71–85, p. 74.

48   Lublin, *Pandora's Box*, 119.

feminism',[49] and Stabile's 'technopragmatism'. All of these terms refer to the biosocial stance regarding issues of sex/gender difference that I advocate. For equivocals, solutions to the dilemmas presented to women by NRTs must be grounded in a methodology that bridges patriarchal binaries including the biology/society distinction. In place of the resisters' 'technophobia' and the embracers' 'technomania', Stabile's proposed 'technopragmatism' insists on the interpenetration of the biological and social realms, the 'bio-social', as the defining character of both *pregnancy* as well as mothering: 'Although feminists must insist that pregnancy is not necessarily synonymous with mothering, they must also insist that both are 'biosocial' experiences – that pregnancy, like mothering occurs within a specific social, economic, cultural, and historical environment and that the experience of pregnancy, as such, is structured by social relations'.[50]

This allows us to resolve the resistance feminists' 'pro-choice but anti-NRTs' dilemma as discussed in the previous chapter. A biosocial view of reproductive justice would require support for those who choose to mother (including through the use of NRTs) and not just support abortion and contraceptive access and rights. On a theoretical level, O'Brien's work founds and continues to sustain a feminist politics of reproduction that does just that. In a sense she applies the spirit of standpoint epistemology, by substituting the gynocentric view of material life based on some 20 years of experience as a midwife to create a view of historical materialism that accounts for women's embodied experience of the world as birthers. Most importantly, her view of reproduction as a thoroughly biosocial process is the paradigm idea that is revitalized in the new material feminisms. In *The Politics of Reproduction* she elucidates how her feminist theory is 'material', because 'it attempts to root this long oppression [of women] in material biological process, rather than in mute, brute biology'.[51]

Like O'Brien's theory, Stabile's proposal is trans-dualistic in attempting to convince one of the falsity of the biological and social distinction of processes considered most 'natural': human reproduction (or pregnancy, childbirth, and nursing). Human reproduction, like bodies, is always already inscribed by social forces because we live within cultures already defined in large part by our techno-social practices, including NRTs. On both a collective and individual level, when,

49   Lublin, *Pandora's Box*, 118. Like the materialist feminisms espoused by Petchesky, MacKinnon, and Colker – for example see Petchesky, 'Foetal Images'; Catherine MacKinnon, *Toward a Feminist Theory of the State*, Boston: Harvard University Press, 1989. Catherine MacKinnon, 'From Practice to Theory, or what Is a White Woman Anyway?', *Yale Journal of Law and Feminism* 4 (1991): 13–22, and Catherine MacKinnon. 'Reflections on Sex Equality under Law', *Yale Law Journal* 100 (1991): 1281–1328; Ruth Colker, 'An Equal Protection Analysis of United States Reproductive Health Policy: Gender, Race, Age, and Class', *Duke Law Journal* (1991): 324–64, and 'The Practice of Theory', *Northwestern University Law Review* 87 (1993): 1273–85.

50   Lublin, *Pandora's Box*, 94.

51   Mary O'Brien, *The Politics of Reproduction*, Boston: Routledge and Kegan Paul, 1981, 44.

how, why, and under what circumstances we get pregnant, gestate and give birth (or not) are matters profoundly circumscribed by inextricably intertwined biological and (techno-)social, or *material*, forces.

Equivocal feminists, as the name suggests, incorporate elements of both embracing and resisting feminists' responses. Their view of women's reproductive control is that it should involve choice guided by certain feminist principles. For them, the only way for women to have control over reproduction is to have choices to do what they see as needed on an individual basis, while prohibiting what is clearly detrimental for the social collective. Also, women are differently socially located and so have different reproductive needs, some of which may require the use of NRTs. The Canadian Royal Commission on New Reproductive Technologies showed that there is no simple formula for deciding which (and whose) principles provide *the* 'feminist' criteria to judge which NRTs are acceptable. The commission's equivocal approach resulted in establishment of a national regulatory body in 2006 and banning of some procedures widely agreed upon by feminists as potentially dangerous for women, such as cloning and those which commercialize reproduction. In the final analysis, however, proceeding 'with care' may be too weak to advance feminist causes which, although diverse, overlap because of women's shared biosocial corporeality.

In many respects the equivocal feminist response to new reproductive technologies, represent the most promising approach to NRTs to bypass the problematic discourses of choice and control and false dualism in general because it entails a biosocial understanding of reproduction. For the same reason, it enables us to address the trans-dualistic negotiations that characterize women's paradoxical embodied existences. The dualism-targeting arguments of the equivocalists is conceptually mirrored in O'Brien's biosocial theory of reproduction, as well as the new feminist materialisms as I explore in the following chapter.

PART III
Material Resolutions

Introduction to Part III

So far I have explored why the body matters regarding NRTs, arguing that women's bodies are a source of their power (albeit a paradoxical one) in patriarchal cultures, and that NRTs disembody women conceptually and physically. By disembodying female reproductive processes, NRTs (and their supporting ideologies), tend to erode women's unique subjectivity (which challenges androcentric hegemony concealed in Western culture), hence their embodied power. I argued that 'the body', in modernity, is linked to subjectivity, agency, and citizenship; and that in the history of Western political thought, authority has been linked to male bodies. The history of the Western world is androcentric, yet based on men's ideological and material appropriation of women's reproductive capacities. The disembodiment wrought by NRTs, when seen as part of a history of birth appropriation in Western thought, reveals the imperative to bring the materiality of bodies, especially reproductive process, back into feminist analysis.

Part III explores 'Material Resolutions' to the bio/social dialectic examined throughout the book. In Chapter 4, I return to Mary O'Brien's complex conception of biosocial reproduction as a mediation of the patriarchal nature/culture dualism, linking her insights to feminist standpoint theory and the new material feminisms as constituting a post-constructionist 'thinking technology'[1] to highlight what the latter enable in feminist thought as a trans-dualist analytic framework. I draw on recent literature which examines the new material feminisms (variously referred to) as part of an emerging multidisciplinary field of scholarship in which feminist theory is prominent, and which begins from a critique of the limits of social constructionism (but also of biological determinism) in favour of a more complex material analysis.

In Chapter 3, I discussed materialism as a way to get at the methodological and worldview aspects of historical materialism and specifically as situated in its socialist feminist appropriation in second wave Anglo-feminism. More specifically I was concerned with materialism as a Marxist methodology of historical materialism adapted within feminism, especially as standpoint epistemology – a concern with social relations as constitutive of subjectivity. In Chapter 4, I will

---

1 Nina Lykke, 'The Timeliness of Post-Constructionism', *NORA – Nordic Journal of Feminist and Gender Research* 18:2 (June 2010): 131–6.

go into the biosocial negotiation associated with O'Brien (1981) and the feminist standpoint epistemology which Nancy Hartsock (1983) developed as the ground for a specifically feminist historical materialism which is implicit in O'Brien's biosocial theory of reproductive consciousness. I am particularly interested in how O'Brien's materialist theory as a feminist standpoint epistemology, maps on to feminist essentialism and anti-essentialism debates, and what role consciousness plays in feminist standpoint and O'Brien's theory.

There are at least three overlapping key dimensions of the biosocial: *methodological* (for example, cartography associated with the trans-disciplinarity of new material feminisms as opposed to linear, more two-dimensional classification); *temporal* in the sense of chronological and teleological relationships, for example modernity as a more or less stable and internally (ideologically) coherent temporal node that precedes postmodernity; and *conceptual*, as in the relationship of ideas over time, and at a time, in complex interrelation for example, what is 'new' about the world in this perspective? But as Nina Lykke and Iris van der Tuin reveal, these are complicated dimensions that can't easily be separated out. However, revisiting O'Brien's reproductive materialist theory, and Hartsock's reflections on her original article in context of its feminist critique, enables us to tease out the significant workings of these interlocking biosocial aspects.

In Chapter 5 and the Conclusion, I outline potential feminist resolutions to a history of patriarchal dualism manifest in birth appropriation by theorizing the 'new' material feminisms as a methodology that is trans-dualistic in the same sense of O'Brien's biosocial reproduction. Chapter 5 frames the new material feminisms as a postconstructionist 'thinking technology', and focuses on what they enable in feminist thought as 'breaking feminist waves' and more broadly, as a trans-disciplinary, trans-dualistic theoretical framework with radical epistemological and methodological potential for addressing disembodying dualism underlying patriarchal praxis. More specifically, I propose that post-constructionism entails a methodology capable of mitigating nature/culture duality in its overlapping but divergent domains; most significantly, in feminist theory, especially the social constructionist/biological essentialist impasse linked to debates about new reproductive technologies.

Chapter 4
Mary O'Bricn and
'The Feminist Standpoint Revisited'

Feminist theorists, going back to the root of theory (*theoria*) are those who engage in 'ways of seeing' the world, particularly by centralizing the role of sex/gender in knowledge practices.[1] The majority do so from the perspective of social epistemology, the philosophical study of the nature of knowledge, that emphasizes the inseparability of individual knowers and communities of knowers. Feminist social epistemology, then, recognizes sex/gender as a feature of embodiment (or corporeally mediated subjectivity) that is always (socially) situated. Embodiment is best understood in contrast to Cartesian dualist theories, based on the mind/body division, which sees the thinking mind as separate from the physical body. As the educational theorist Grumet wrote, '"it is not I think therefore I am", rather it is because I am embodied and situated that I think in particular ways'.[2]

The feminist approach to the phenomenology of embodiment has a long history that both engages but moves beyond the mind/body debate which is variously manifest, but often as disputes over the extent to which embodied sex/gender is experienced as socioculturally constructed, hence changeable, as opposed to biologically limiting. It also involves feminist epistemologies, especially feminist standpoint theory, that tackles the complicated relationship of bodies, selves and subjectivities, in addition to that of sex/gender. This chapter concerns questions of feminist epistemology that emphasize materiality as a complex biosocial process associated with Mary O'Brien's dialectical reproductive materialism, especially as a feminist standpoint epistemology in the tradition of Nancy Hartsock. I am particularly interested in how O'Brien's materialist theory as a kind of feminist standpoint epistemology maps onto feminist essentialism/constructionism debates, and what role consciousness plays in O'Brien's theory and feminist standpoint epistemology.

Mary O'Brien's Dialectical Reproductive Materialism

Mary O'Brien developed a dialectical analysis of reproductive process by adapting Marx's method of historical materialism and Hegel's notion of dialectics, while

---

1 'Feminist Social Epistemology', *Stanford Encyclopedia of Philosophy*, Stanford University, 2006, Web.

2 Cited in Annabelle Mooney and Betsy Evans, *Globalization: The Key Concepts*, London: Routledge, 2007, 76.

including reproductive process and labour which both assigned to biological nature hence excluded as involuntary and part of 'necessity'. Dialectics refers to 'the method of reasoning which aims to understand things concretely in all their movement, change and interconnection, with their opposite and contradictory sides in unity'.[3] This complex, dynamic negotiation, borrowed from Hegel, informs Marx's theory of dialectical (or historical) materialism as both a theory of history, and a revolutionary political principle. The result of O'Brien's integration of reproductive process and dialectical materialism is a thoroughly dialectical understanding of reproduction as the substructure of history.[4] In O'Brien's analysis, biological processes are not fixed but dialectical and historical, hence Jeff Hearne's description of her methodology as 'reproductive dialectical materialism'.[5]

O'Brien's materialism is distinguished from Marxist materialism in key ways. First, she applies her analysis to reproduction as dialectical in itself and with reference to processes of production; second, she assigns theoretical, epistemological, and ontological primacy to the relations of reproduction (or procreation of the species) as opposed to the daily reproduction of the individual; and finally in that she understands materialism itself as fundamentally dialectical. Anticipating the new material feminisms O'Brien believed, '[t]he "material" realm – biological nature comprehended in human thought and practice – is itself dialectically structured'.[6] In *The Politics of Reproduction* she elucidates how her feminist theory is 'material', because 'it attempts to root this long oppression [of women] in material biological process, rather than in mute, brute biology'.[7] Men attempting to appropriate the products of birth from which they are alienated, not brute biology, is the root of male dominance. That is, biology itself is a complex biosocial process rather than a thing, but a process (nonetheless) defined in androcentric terms in patriarchal cultures.[8] For her, giving birth, which is a uniquely female process, is historical in that it is the integration of consciousness and knowing on the one hand, and of action on the other. Although birth is involuntary it is also constituted of specific knowledge and awareness and is constitutive of a particular subjectivity and culture that is naturally only that of biological women.

O'Brien draws from Gramsci to talk about patriarchal hegemony, since she believes his analysis provides an escape from the economic determinism of orthodox Marxism. She appropriates his understanding of civil society as a

---

3   Glossary of Terms, 'Dialectics', *Encyclopedia of Marxism*, Marxist Internet Archive, 1999, Web.

4   Nancy Hartsock, 'Mary O'Brien's Contributions to Contemporary Feminist Theory', *Canadian Woman Studies* 18:4 (1999): 62.

5   Jeff Hearne, 'Mary O'Brien … Certainly the Most Important Single Intellectual Influence … ', *Canadian Woman Studies*, 18:4 (Winter 1999): 15.

6   Mary O'Brien, *The Politics of Reproduction*, Boston: Routledge and Kegan Paul, 1981.

7   O'Brien, *The Politics of Reproduction*, 44.

8   O'Brien, *The Politics of Reproduction*, 231.

mediator between state and economy and theorizes that the development of consent for patriarchal praxis was embedded in this realm of civil society under which reproductive process falls.[9] The result of her integration of reproductive process and historical materialism is a thoroughly dialectical understanding of male and female reproductive consciousnesses, which in spite of its nuance and relevance to ongoing questions of gendered subjectivities, has often been misunderstood and dismissed as essentialist.

She recognized the possibility of agency in the spaces between production and reproduction in dialectical relationship, constituting a neo Marxist approach to the relationship of base and superstructure. 'This profound restructuring of base and superstructure is what O'Brien calls "the philosophy of birth" and "part of but separate from the historical movement of class struggle"'.[10] O'Brien's work is socialist feminist in renegotiating orthodox Marxist understandings of relationships between production and reproduction, and of the meaning of biology and women's specific historical associations with it in Western systems of patriarchy. Women's reproduction gives rise to particular gendered subjectivity – men's and women's reproductive consciousnesses – regardless of whether individual women reproduce or individual men nurture and care for babies and children. For example, we do not have to use IVF to be affected by the technomaterial and cultural disembodiment of reproduction that follows from new reproductive technologies.

O'Brien's brand of dialectics also believes historical process, as related both to production *and* reproduction, is comprised of 'a series of alienations, contradictions and mediation'.[11] For example the distinction between public and private spheres is a tangible manifestation of the attempted containment of productive and reproductive process, but the dialectical character of the two continually emerges in issues like prostitution, pornography, worker's health and other junctures of individual and species needs. It also emerges clearly in the commodification of reproduction in conceptive technologies (such as debates over stem cells, egg donation, and surrogacy highlight) which O'Brien recognized as rendering 'the relationship between capitalism and patriarchy fecund',[12] though she was most concerned with contraception.[13] But it was her student Somer Brodribb who did most to explain this relationship, first reading reproductive consciousness into new

---

9   Lerner, *The Creation of Patriarchy*, New York: Oxford University Press, 1986.

10   O'Brien, *The Politics of Reproduction*, 7; Burfoot, Annette, 'In-Appropriation – A Critique of "Proceed with Care: Final Report of the Royal Commission on New Reproductive Technologies"', *Women's Studies International Forum* 18:4 (1995).

11   Mary O'Brien, 'Feminist Theory and Dialectical Logic', in *Feminist Theory: A Critique of Ideology*, ed. Nannerl O. Keohane, Michelle Z. Rosaldo and Barbara C. Gelpi, Chicago: University of Chicago Press, 1982, 99–112.

12   Mary O'Brien, 'State Power and Reproductive Freedom', *Canadian Woman Studies* 18:4 (Winter 1999): 79–85.

13   O'Brien, *The Politics of Reproduction*, 158–9; O'Brien, 'State Power and Reproductive Freedom', 81.

reproductive technologies and their legal and other ramifications in the 1980s. Conceptive technologies do create a sort of 'consumer choice in childbirth' (at least in theory) which can be positive in terms both individual and collective as explored in Chapter 1, but they also exacerbate, and individualize current unequal gendered reproductive relations.[14] Annette Burfoot's application of Bauman's concept of liquidity to reproductive technology highlights that reproduction, like other issues of great social and political significance is subject to the entrenched, if changeable, logic of global capitalism, including individualism, and so has become difficult to articulate as a social issue. But reproduction is a political issue that requires collective action, in addition to private decision making.

O'Brien's insights about men's 'second natures' as coming from their mediation of reproductive experiences (of alienation) are unique and widely recognized in feminist studies. That this way of seeing the world effects a masculinist denial of birth, or 'first nature', evident in a death impulse is attributed to Brodribb who effectively traces such in the denial of matter (considered the feminine principle) and its significance by comparison to form (presented as a masculine principle) from Classical Greek texts through to postmodern psychoanalysis.[15] Furthermore, Burfoot employs O'Brien's analysis to contemporary forms of reproductive technology representing a contemporary socialist feminist use of O'Brien's dialectical reproductive materialism in light of recent developments in egg donation and surrogacy.

Especially pertinent to the paradox of reproduction, or women's embodied reproductive experiences as a source of both profound power and vulnerability is O'Brien's conceptualization of the two moments of significant change in reproductive process. These 'moments' were, first, the discovery of physiological paternity, which made clear the male's role in unmediated reproductive process – a dialectical situation in which the man is alienated from his offspring and hence from species continuity and a sense of continuity over time – and second, the development of reliable and widespread contraceptive technology which permits the separation of sexual intercourse and reproduction for women, as for men, which results in women's self-alienation from reproductive process. The first gave rise to various forms of mediation of the alienation of his reproductive process, for example, the establishment of both public and private infrastructures to ensure the fidelity of women, specifically the ownership of particular women's sexual and reproductive services. The most obvious of these is the institution of the patriarchal nuclear family in contractual marriage.[16] The second is the advent of mass contraceptive technology.

For her, contraceptive technology signifies great change in the social relations of reproduction, if it exists on a mass scale, since it allows women to separate

---

14   Somer Brodribb, *Nothing Mat(t)ers: A Feminist Critique of Postmodernism*, Toronto: James Lorimer and Company, 1993.

15   Brodribb, *Nothing Mat(t)ers*.

16   See also Lerner, *The Creation of Patriarchy*.

heterosexual intercourse and reproduction for the first time: an experience that without technology is only men's. Contraceptives go back to pre-Christian Egypt; the difference from modern contraception is its mass production, distribution, and control by men through the medical industrial complex. For O'Brien, contraceptive technology alienates women and their reproductive processes, which must then be mediated as for men. This entails a change in women's experience of reproduction, in its overlapping biological (separating sex from reproduction), psychological (recognition of choice, self-value, sexual identity and agency) and sociocultural dimensions (behaviour vis-à-vis potential sex partners, not just co-parents). This new development allows for rationalization of reproduction including the scientization of birth by male scientists with which the resistors were concerned. However, it also allows women, and men, to control the process that provides the material basis for the structuring of social, political, and cultural life.

O'Brien believed that mass contraceptive technology had the promise of liberating women, not just of furthering control over women's reproduction by men. This is largely because '[i]n the first place, it provides a heretofore non-existent material base for gender equality, rescuing the notion of equality from the dubious justifications of rhetoric and placing it firmly on a material basis'.[17] Before the advent of mass contraception, the only way to choose parenthood was to be celibate or non-heterosexual. This is also why, she explains, it constitutes in Hegel's terms, a 'world-historical event' nonetheless, since she nowhere specifies that she is dealing with geographic limits, we must assume that she meant her theory to apply universally. In contrast, I explore the Anglo-American component of the affluent North/West, and this particular model of birth appropriation as it has developed and been applied there. But patriarchy and male dominance exist outside the West, although the specificities of these and other non-Western reproductive dialectics are beyond the scope of this book.

According to O'Brien, the uncertainty of paternity leads to men creating institutions to mediate generational change. She claims that 'paternity is essentially idealist' since it is not a direct and material experience and requires the rationalization of a 'cause and effect' relationship. Women's reproductive consciousnesses, on the other hand, because mothers usually know their children, share the integration of historical and cyclical time (imparting a sense of continuity over time).[18] Maternity, unlike paternity, has an experienced material basis; if conscious during labour, no biological mother need wonder if the child she bears is her own. Through technology, paternity now has a material base in DNA testing, but the uncertainty of fatherhood requires either technology or restrictions on women's freedom to mediate it.[19]

---

17   O'Brien, 'Feminist Theory and Dialectical Logic', 110.

18   Frieda Johles Forman and Caoran Sowton, eds, *Taking our Time: Feminist Perspectives on Temporality*, Oxford: Pergamon Press, 1989; Heather Menzies, 'Technological Time and Infertility', *Canadian Woman Studies* 18:4 (1999): 69–74.

19   Brodribb, *Nothing Mat(t)ers*.

O'Brien never resolved the contentions and quarrels that surrounded her radical theory, especially as they reveal deeply complicated conflicts between anti-natal and pro-natal positions and historical differences between mainstream Western women and Third World and minority women. Most significantly, her universalist claims were denounced as essentialist, as was her seemingly heterosexual bias because of her use of 'sex' to mean heterosexual intercourse. But as Burfoot claims 'On re-reading O'Brien after years of teaching postmodern social theory, I am struck by her epistemological self-reflexivity as she acknowledges that "feminist theory has to be biased because it is anti-bias"'.[20] Hartsock similarly lauded O'Brien for reminding feminists that 'the view from the margins' is also 'the view from below'. O'Brien's is an unapologetic view of women's reproduction as challenging the production/reproduction and nature/culture dichotomies.[21] Hartsock reads in O'Brien an elaborate and 'nuanced' account of [her own] feminist standpoint theory, providing a qualified endorsement: 'It is important to read her work for the methodology it embraces rather than for the specific categories she puts forward'.[22] By contrast, Burfoot suggests that O'Brien's feminist ideas anticipate postmodern theorization but it is the standpoint dimensions of her work – imbricated in the feminist social constructionist/biological essentialist impasse that was the stumbling block for her uptake.[23]

Regardless of one's perception of O'Brien's work, it is a way of assessing the changing material and ideological structure of reproductive process that has outlived its original focus. Gestational surrogacy is exemplary of how women's unique reproductive labour continues to get lost in the Marxist frameworks rooted in men's productive labour, for example the privileging of the genetic contribution in surrogacy arrangements. When gestating and birthing children is separated from and pitted against genetic contribution as the *sine qua non* of kinship relations, we have to question the epistemological roots of such assumptions in unqualified hegemonic androcentrism. For example, Somer Brodribb in reference to the Ontario Law Reform Commission Report writes, 'The all-male commission stresses that the mother's importance to the child is merely genetic, and ignores the centrality of birthing, which has traditionally established a woman's relationship to a child'.[24]

---

20   Annette Burfoot, 'Revisiting Mary O'Brien – Reproductive Consciousness and Liquid Maternity', Marxisms and Feminisms on the Edge, Society for Socialist Studies: Annual Meeting. Victoria, BC, 5–7 June 2013. Paper Presentation.

21   Nancy Hartsock, 'Mary O'Brien's Contributions', 67.

22   Nancy Hartsock, *The Feminist Standpoint Revisited & Other Essays*, Boulder, CO: Westview Press, 1998, 66.

23   See especially Burfoot, 'Revisiting Mary O'Brien', but also Jean-Francois Lyotard, 'Introduction to The Postmodern Condition: A Report on Knowledge', in *Twentieth Century Political Theory: A Reader*, ed. Stephen Eric Bronner, New York: Routledge, 1997, 239–41.

24   Somer Brodribb, 'Off the Pedestal and onto the Block? Motherhood, Reproductive Technologies, and the Canadian State', *Canadian Journal of Women and the Law* 1:2 (1986): 420.

O'Brien's feminist materialist theory is a necessary starting point and rich resource for understanding and negotiating the lived complexity of Western patriarchal cultures and is evident, for example, in the biosocial negotiations of the equivocal feminist responses to NRTs. If we can see past the dated discourse, an unavoidable but superficial artifact of academic trends, her complex understanding of the relationship of ideas, society and biology in reproduction (or consciousness, social relations, and biological process in her terms), is relevant and critical to the feminist movement today, and indeed to the unresolved nature/ nurture (or sex/gender) tension in Western culture more broadly. Ultimately, her focus on women's reproductive commonality is sorely needed in contemporary feminist theory, especially when it is paired with a substantive understanding of diversity and difference and genuine strategies to address intersectionality, or the way multiple social location fundamentally defines one's experience of reproductive consciousness.

O'Brien may not have framed her contribution in terms of feminist epistemology generally, nor of standpoint epistemologically specifically, but her work implicitly proposes a specific standpoint from men's and women's differing reproductive consciousnesses, as Hartsock recognizes: 'Her argument for a superior understanding which has not had power is more nuanced than my own in my feminist standpoint essay, but the impulse and conclusion are similar'.[25] Although O'Brien's standpoint is implicit and assumed as Hartsock pointed out, and rests on differential reproductive consciousnesses it could be seen as a *women's* standpoint rather than a *feminist* standpoint, which was Hartsock's purview. What is certain is O'Brien's unapologetically counter-hegemonic view is thoroughly dialectically materialist in the Marxist sense that things do not 'exist outside of or prior to the processes, flows, and relations that create, sustain, or undermine them'.[26] O'Brien retains this centrally important and contemporarily relevant insight but her theory of reproductive consciousness is biosocial, that is, it underscores biological materiality as an undeniable agent of such social and historical process.

Revisiting 'The Feminist Standpoint Revisited'

Feminist political theorist Nancy Hartsock was the first to develop feminist standpoint theory (1983) but standpoint became an established category of feminist epistemology as set out in Sandra Harding's *The Science Question in Feminism* (1986) which launched the now classic tripartite classification of feminist empiricism, feminist standpoint epistemology, and feminist post-modernism. Although the original categories, have been modified and even

---

25   Hartsock, 'Mary O'Brien's Contributions', 66.
26   David Harvey, *Justice, Nature, and the Geography of Difference*, New York: Blackwell, 1996 cited in Hartsock, 'Mary O'Brien's Contributions', 64.

improved (by Lykke in particular), Harding's concepts remain foundational in feminist studies.[27] Feminist empiricism seeks (as a basis for better science) to incorporate women's observable and measurable experiences into the implicitly androcentric Western scientific model. In contrast feminist post-modernism expresses skepticism about identity hence the validity of rooting knowledge in experiences based on false (and totalizing) categories, like 'women', but feminist standpoint which differs from a generic 'women's perspective' was to be epistemically privileged for Harding because it entailed the political engagement of feminists and a corresponding critical consciousness.[28] However, as feminist epistemologies proliferated and evolved most actively in 1980s and early 1990s, Harding's typology was challenged and 'cross-fertiliz[ed]' and she has framed her own position as a blend of standpoint theory and feminist postmodernism.[29]

My focus is the biosocial dialectic at play in Hartsock's standpoint theory as a major category of feminist epistemology (which may be on the cusp of a renaissance in post-constructionism.) Standpoint is about 'epistemic advantage' but as a social epistemology, also situated knowledges and multiple subjectivities.[30] In fact, they cannot be separated, as the epistemic advantage of the feminist standpoint is only possible as a consequence of the other two dimensions. Standpoint comes about through the recognition of more than one view of the world, which originates in a discord or misfit between one's own experience and the mainstream discourse about the world. This can, in theory, lead to the more complex and broader understanding of situated knowledges and multiple subjectivities, and a critical epistemology. This view contradicts the major critique of standpoint theory as universalist narrative based on a sex-linked essentialism, but Hartsock's response to such critiques, especially in her reflection on the original argument 15 years after its publication, enable us to get deeper into the biosocial negotiation relevant to feminist studies from O'Brien, through Hartsock to the new material feminisms.

In brief, feminist standpoint is a development upon Marxist theorist Georg Lukac's privileging of the proletariat's oppression as a dual vision, giving rise to a liberatory working class consciousness. As such, sex (in Hartsock's terms) is substituted for proletariat oppression as a potential revolutionary source of awareness and she formulated the work as a 'ground for a specifically feminist historical materialism'. It is because of a focus on women as a category (seen to be universal and culturally transcendent) because of her use of sex, rather than gender, that it has been a source of various interpretations and critique, if

---

27   Hartsock, *The Feminist Standpoint Revisited.*

28   'Feminist Social Epistemology', *Stanford Encyclopedia of Philosophy.*

29   'Feminist Social Epistemology', *Stanford Encyclopedia of Philosophy*; Sandra Harding, *Whose Science? Whose Knowledge?*, Milton Keynes: Open University Press, 1991.

30   Kristina Rolin, 'The Bias Paradox in Feminist Standpoint Epistemology', *Episteme: A Journal of Social Epistemology* 3:1 (2006): 125–36.

also fruitful feminist debate.[31] Standpoint theory has been widely interpreted and employed, and Hartsock distances her feminist standpoint theory from more general standpoint theories.

The central argument of feminist standpoint epistemology is an appropriation of Marxist dialectical materialism, so entails the working out of the biology/society dualism in that particular approach. It is often the assumption of a biologically essentialized understanding of women as underlying standpoint theory, and similar reductionism in Marx's theory that informs critique of Hartsock's original concept. But there is good reason to believe that though not faultless, Hartsock's feminist standpoint was not essentialist. For example she admits, that her 'too-literal reading of Marx's own too-schematic two-class model of society' was reductionist in her focus on women as a group similarly oppressed under patriarchal capitalism, and so did not account for the complex and divergent experiences of individual women.[32]

Furthermore, feminist standpoint epistemology occupies an unclear position vis-à-vis Marxist materialism as a function of its uneasy, paradoxical status as both part of Enlightenment humanism (as a scientific approach) and a fundamental challenge to its liberal individualism. These ambiguities may be explained by the way that feminist standpoint epistemology is the result of the feminist appropriation of Marxist concepts that do not fit perfectly, so entail subtle negotiations and experiments. They also cannot be separated from imbrication in particular (boundary) disputes amongst Marxist and radical feminism synthesized but not wholly resolved in socialist feminism. This is clear in the way materialism can be attributed to each of these, in some ways similar, but also quite diverse approaches. Its hybrid status implies fusion which leaves seams that have the dual character of weakness, in terms of proneness to breakage, but can also be understood as nodes of flexibility and possibility.

Also part of the essentialist critique of standpoint theory is the latter's assumed romanticization of 'the view from below', but there is a difference between standpoint as an 'achieved stance' or technique, and a point of view. Hartsock's theory advocates a feminist standpoint, rather than a women's perspective; the former is won by struggle and activity conscious of complicity and complexity in multiple (and even contradictory) consciousnesses.[33] Although standpoint privileges the epistemic position of the oppressed insofar as it can give rise to an improved, counterhegemonic not just a different kind of knowledge, it does not essentialize the source of such awareness. As Harding clarifies, 'standpoint theory does not require feminine essentialism but rather analyses the essentialism that androcentrism attributes to women; nor does it assume that women are free

---

31   Hartsock, *The Feminist Standpoint Revisited*, 230.

32   Hartsock, *The Feminist Standpoint Revisited*.

33   For further discussion of this idea, see Carl Marzani, *The Open Marxism of Antonio Gramsci*, trans. C. Marzani, New York: Cameron Associates.

of participation in racist, classist, or homophobic social relations'.[34] 'Rather it is to note that marginalized groups are less likely to mistake themselves for the universal "man"'.[35]

Following from the sentimentalization of an underclass in Marxist-inspired standpoint theories is assumptions about the notion of women's critical consciousness as essentialist, not unlike in critiques of O'Brien's reproductive consciousness. Hartsock addressed the claims she (and O'Brien) were similarly biologically determinist – emphasizing misunderstandings of Marx's more subtle than recognized biosocial dynamic in dialectical materialism. This is addressed in Hartsock's explanation that in her use of sex rather than gender, she meant to imply nature as never outside sociality in Marx's sense. The claims that her work was essentialist stem from a lack of familiarity with this fundamental Marxist principle; there may be no outside to 'nature' in Marxist theory, but such nature is fundamentally social and historical – that is, our nature is social process. Recognizing her use of 'sex' rather than 'gender' did not work, she goes further to reflect; 'in a sense it could not work, given the terms of debate at that time ... I can still think of no terminology that refuses the opposition between nature and culture in the context of contemporary US feminist theory'. This is changing with the post-constructionist new material feminisms, as Lykke's useful terms highlight and I will explore. 'But what I was attempting to do was to denaturalize nature (Haraway's phrase) and to refuse the split'.[36] The same can be said of O'Brien's reproductive materialism, and this reinforces the need for a revisitation, and a hermeneutic reading of centrally important texts.

Hartsock's work in 'The Feminist Standpoint Revisited' involved a revision to her original theory, most significantly one that anticipates newer materialisms such as Lykke describes in feminist postconstructionism, in that it is not a feminist standpoint, but feminist *standpoints* based in Donna Haraway's situated knowledges.[37] Harstock names Paula Moya's 'realist theory of Chicana identity' as a detailed account of the process by which standpoints emerge because it involves overlapped racial, sexual, and sex/gendered memberships. Further she reiterates the achieved character of a standpoint, in that 'a standpoint is constituted by more than oppression and cannot be reduced to identity politics as usually understood' because it's not an individualist theory but about social collectives/ivities which are in part 'formed by their oppression and marginalization'[38] hence have a common base of experience if differentiated individual experiences. Hartsock is concerned with 'doubled or multiple consciousness of oppressed groups',[39] not a universal consciousness because, she emphasizes, her concepts are specific and about social

---

34   Hartsock, *The Feminist Standpoint Revisited*, 233.
35   Hartsock, *The Feminist Standpoint Revisited*, 236.
36   Hartsock, 'Mary O'Brien's Contributions', 235.
37   Hartsock, *The Feminist Standpoint Revisited*, 236.
38   Hartsock, *The Feminist Standpoint Revisited*, 239–41.
39   Hartsock, *The Feminist Standpoint Revisited*, 233.

rather than individual relations. Since her argument is predominantly concerned with 'the theoretical conditions of possibility for creating alternatives' it is not meant as an accurate diagnosis of actual (individual) women's consciousnesses. Importantly, she credits Haraway as a key example of standpoint theory in this regard.[40]

Furthermore, Hartsock's revised standpointism has much in common with Haraway's notion of situated knowledges and the 'multiple subjectivities' aspects of standpoint. Although many feminist theorists have been considered standpoint theorists (like O'Brien), Haraway is one that Hartsock considers a standpoint theorist, although she is not typically categorized as such.[41] This is because the situated knowledges she fleshes out 'as the knowledges of the dominated are 'savvy to modes of denial', which include repression, forgetting, and disappearing. Thus, while recognizing themselves as never fixed or fully achieved, they can claim to present a truer, or more adequate account of reality'.[42] She emphasizes that the features of the multiple subjectivities she advocates are both specific and yet common and shared positionalities.[43] In Lykke's theorization, however, Hartsock's classic feminist standpoint theory is at odds with interesectionality largely because of the former's metanarrative contribution, and the latter's deconstruction of the same. Hartsock similarly positioned her standpointism as a necessary counterpoint to postmodern epistemology and as Lykke clarified, this is because postmodernism actually constitutes an anti-epistemology rather than an epistemological framework. Lykke then goes on to resolve this gap claiming, 'notions such as mobility and multiplicity, on the one hand, and situatedness and localization, on the other' which 'might seem contradictory, do not need to be seen as mutually exclusive'. Various feminisms have worked with and beyond feminist standpoint in light of its weaknesses especially in light of postmodern critiques associated with intersectional difference, and the dangers of metanarrative.[44]

Since a standpoint is implicated in a process involving critical awareness of difference and its political and epistemic implications, it is linked to the other claim of standpoint theory that such knowledge is 'less partial and distorted, and hence more objective'.[45] This is a new kind of objectivity associated with Haraway in the history of feminist science and technology studies whereby objective does not mean the view from nowhere, but the critical awareness of the view from as many somewheres (especially marginal ones) as possible. Hence objectivity takes on a democratic dimension, and is seen as 'social process' whereby the inclusion of as much diverse experience (not just interests or values *per se*) as possible is a

---

40   Hartsock, *The Feminist Standpoint Revisited*, 236.

41   Hartsock, *The Feminist Standpoint Revisited*, 228.

42   Hartsock, *The Feminist Standpoint Revisited*, 244–5.

43   Hartsock, *The Feminist Standpoint Revisited*, 244.

44   Nina Lykke, *Feminist Studies: A Guide to Intersectional Theory, Methodology, and Writing*, New York: Routledge, 2010.

45   'Feminist Social Epistemology', *Stanford Encyclopedia of Philosophy*.

fundamental feature of reliable knowledge.[46] This is where the ethical and political aspects of the epistemological come into view. Knowing as a social practice rather than a purely solitary activity which happens through engagement with others requires ethical accountability. Barad's 'ethico-epistem-ontology' is a shorthand, for this rather complex idea. There is, in fact, a 'complex network of epistemic relations between knowers' which requires us all, especially those engaged in research and knowledge production to take responsibility for patterns of ignorance and illumination of some ways of knowing and not others (as per Haraway).[47]

Conclusion

Feminist standpoint theory represents a negotiation of the two seemingly radically divergent traditions of Marxist (hence modern) and postmodern political theory. Feminist standpoint as Hartsock's 'ground for a specifically feminist historical materialism' conveys an ongoing commitment to Marxist materialist methods and principles, but it also incorporated a postmodern understanding that accommodates multiple differences especially in its later formulations. As a socialist feminist innovation, standpoint epistemology is unsurprisingly a synthesis of seemingly divergent foci on patriarchy, economic class and psychoanalytic/postmodern ideas (about subjectivity) as well. Standpoint epistemology evolved in the history of socialist feminism during the period when it incorporated a psychoanalytic approach within its materialist analysis (especially regarding Mitchell's *Women: The Longest Revolution* (1966) and the famous insights of Gilligan (1982) and Chodorow (1978). In this view, post-structuralist materialism deepens the social constructionist elements of Marxist variants by focusing on the process of materialization. Standpoint theory inherits this counter-intuitive hybridity of Marxist/modern concerns with social structures and historical change/process, and a post-structuralist focus on the discursive process by which we come to embody social location.

Feminist studies of science and technology scholars from across wide-ranging disciplines like political philosopher Sonia Kruks, and feminist quantum physicist Barad have noted the connections between different materialist traditions – as indeed Zalewski prefigured in linking 'modern' and 'postmodern' approaches within feminism more generally.[48] Kruks discusses the overlaps of various 'genres' of materialism in this proposed materialist renaissance showing how the post-structuralist and the neo-Marxist variants are linked in their emphasis on 'the

---

46   'Feminist Social Epistemology', *Stanford Encyclopedia of Philosophy*.

47   Karen Barad, *Meeting the Universe Halfway: Quantum Physics and the Entanglement of Matter and Meaning*, Durham, NC and London: Duke University Press, 2007, 23.

48   See Marysia Zalewski, *Feminism after Postmodernism: Theorising Through Practice*, London and New York: Routledge, 2000.

ways in which subjectivity arises as the reflex or expression of social practices, or as the effect of discourses'.[49] In my terms they are both constructionist at base, or in Elizabeth Grosz's phrasing they work 'from the outside in' instead of 'the inside out'.[50]

We can examine the tensions between postmodern and Marxist materialism in spite of their common constructionist approach, as playing out in the new post-constructionist materialisms. 'Gender de/constructionism' is Lykke's umbrella term that encompasses theories that are determinist on both sides of the biology/society dichotomy (encompassing both Marxist and postmodern types of constructionism as I have examined them) whereas 'corpomaterialist' feminist theories are post-constructionist in the sense of critical of 'tendencies in feminist gender de/constructionism to focus on historical-sociocultural and/or linguistic-discursive gender constructions as being detached from sexed embodiment and from the materiality of bodies'.[51] Their emphasis on materiality focuses on the agency of biology while avoiding biological determinism. A continuation of Hartsock's project, Lykke's innovation is '*an updated and revised version of standpoint epistemology* that, in line with the feminist debate on *intersectionality*, addresses the question of how to articulate the standpoint of the knower, understood as a multiply located subject of research'.[52] Starting from Harding's tripartite theory of feminist epistemologies, Lykke revises feminist postmodernism to 'postmodern anti-epistemologies' because rather than positing new epistemologies, they highlight the 'hidden gender-conservative effects' of all foundational theories, even ones that appear radical. Furthermore, she adds a fourth category, 'post-constructionist feminist epistemologies'. This addition enables the examination of those feminist epistemologies that both take account of postmodern anti-epistemologies and yet go beyond to affirm embodied ('corpomaterialist') material 'as starting points for epistemological reflections'.[53]

Van der Tuin grapples with categorizing the new material feminisms, ultimately landing on the trope of generation which plays on the notion of inheritance without the teleological connotation. The new material feminisms inherited feminist standpoint theory (hence engage with historical materialism) and the new materialists 'claim that a fruitful feminist positioning entails a focus on the material-semiotic (neither solely nature nor solely culture.)'[54] Furthermore,

---

49   Sonia Kruks, 'Simone de Beauvoir: Engaging Discrepant Materialisms', in *New Materialisms: Ontology, Agency and Poltics*, ed. Diana Coole and Samantha Frost, Durham, NC: Duke University Press, 2010, 259.

50   Cited in Kruks, 'Simone de Beauvoir', 259.

51   Lykke, *Feminist Studies*, 203.

52   Lykke, *Feminist Studies*, 126–7.

53   Lykke, *Feminist Studies*, 10.

54   Iris Van der Tuin, 'Deflationary Logic: Response to Sara Ahmed's "Imaginary Prohibitions: Some Preliminary Remarks on the Founding Gestures of the "New Materialism"'", *European Journal of Women's Studies* 15:4 (2008) 414–15.

what she calls the 'new materialism' constitutes a 'feminist epistemic realm' that engages with but is not simply proposing 'a (historical) materialism 'proper'' and uncritical feminist standpoint theory redux, nor past feminist biologies. Instead, 'What we find here is feminist generation'.[55] Van der Tuin is anti-dialectical in advocating the bridging rather than 'sequential negation' of distinct approaches and categories because the latter subverts teleological progression narrative and credits the new materialisms with achieving this.

Van der Tuin's extensive theory cannot be fully expounded here, but by feminist generation she means that new materialism breaks out of the linear and teleological classification of feminist epistemologies/waves. This is better than compartmentalizing feminist ideas in a historical and ideological sense. 'The shared conversation of new materialism defines generationality as generative; generative of shared feminist conversations between Third-wave feminist epistemologists from different inter-disciplines, and between third- [like Rosi Braidotti] and second- wave [like Harding and Jaggar] feminist epistemologists'.[56] Braidotti is categorized as such because she is non-dialectical, non-linear and non-teleological in approach to feminist epistemology and its generationality.[57] She is also credited with coining the phrase 'new materialism' as 'a more radical sense of materialism' by framing it as '[r]ethinking the embodied structure of human subjectivity after Foucault'.[58]

The complex negotiations of the biosocial dialectic in O'Brien's reproductive materialism which constitutes an implicit standpoint epistemology are apparent in a vibrant and growing literature and approach in feminist theory somewhat controversially announcing a 'material turn' but safely categorized under Lykke's umbrella term, 'post-constructionism'.[59] Lykke's complex theorization bridges standpoint theory as an onto-epistemological innovation that carries us from Hartsock to the new material feminisms. 'As is the case in Marxist epistemology, a feminist standpoint epistemology is linked up with a certain ontological starting point in a social theory (a feminist materialist theory of society)'.[60] The difference with post-constructionist feminist epistemology (in Lykke's account) is 'They are not anti-epistemological, but base themselves firmly in alternative epistemological approaches' claiming the importance of being 'able to speak about the world as a pre-discursive facticity endowed with a non-determinist, but independent agency'.[61]

---

55   Van der Tuin, 'Deflationary Logic'.

56   Iris Van der Tuin, '"Jumping Generations": On Second- and Third-wave Feminist Epistemology', *Australian Feminist Studies* 24:59 (2009): 28.

57   Van der Tuin, 'Jumping Generations', 18.

58   Rosi Braidotti, '"Teratologies"', in *Deleuze and Feminist Theory*, ed. Ian Buchanan Claire Colebrook, Edinburgh: Edinburgh University Press, 2000 cited in Iris Van der Tuin and Rick Dolphijn, 'The Transversality New Materialism', *Women: A Cultural Review* 21:2 (2010): 166–7.

59   Nina Lykke, 'The Timeliness of Post-Constructionism', *NORA – Nordic Journal of Feminist and Gender Research* 18:2 (June 2010): 131–6.

60   Lykke, *Feminist Studies*, 206.

61   Lykke, *Feminist Studies*, 209.

In the next chapter I investigate post-constructionism as a potential next step in biosocial negotiations, started in feminist standpoint epistemology but leading to a breaking feminist waves methodology in feminist theory. Rather than a teleological investigation, it is part of a continuous working out of the relationship of biology and society in social and political theory and emerging in feminist studies. The common element across materialisms before the postconstructionist turn, was a concern with the features of individual embodiment and social location, and the process of social inscription as the starting point of analysis rather than biological essence. It is because of this that older materialisms, even with the incorporation of especially postmodern theory, remained mired in social constructionism. While postmodern theories aimed to add agency to the modern/Marxist structuralist debate, they ultimately failed because they remained over-reliant on a dualistic anti-essentialism in its emphasis on discursive materialization. Van der Tuin and Dolphijn argue, 'New materialism is a cultural theory for the twenty-first century that attempts to show how postmodern cultural theory, while claiming otherwise, has made use of a conceptualization of "post" that is dualist'.[62] However, tempting it is to place new material feminisms as a straightforward synthesis/resolution of the failings of postmodernism and Marxist materialisms, what new material feminisms offer is fundamentally undermined in such a depiction as I explore in the following chapter.[63]

---

62   Van der Tuin and Dolphijn, 'The Transversality of New Materialism', 166–7.

63   Van der Tuin and Dolphijn, 'The Transversality of New Materialism'. See also Kruks, 'Simone de Beauvoir'.

Chapter 5

Postconstructionist, 'New' Material Feminisms: Breaking Feminist Waves

The new material feminisms as a significant manifestation of the biosocial negotiations explored in relation to Mary O'Brien and feminist standpoint epistemology also represent a fundamentally and thoroughly trans-dual methodology that collapses the modern/postmodern dichotomy in its various linear and teleological manifestations. As Iris van der Tuin and Rick Dolphijn succinctly put it, 'New materialism is a cultural theory for the twenty-first century ... that is non-foundationalist yet non-relativist'.[1] As such it is promising as a method to transcend seemingly irreconcilable differences associated with the entrenched modern/postmodern division within feminism, most often understood as a (biologically) essentialist/(social) constructionist impasse. It is an impasse because this debate is generally characterized by a deeply entrenched conservatism whereby biology and culture are presented as opposed positions leaving us at a stalemate regarding 'the woman question' which remains foundational to movements for sex/gender equality however conceived or identified.

As explored in the last chapter, assigning the new material feminisms to a particular temporal and theoretical location is important insofar as its heterogeneity serves to indicate the common ground of many otherwise diverse (even antagonistic) theoretical traditions.[2] Here I elaborate on that theme in teasing out further methodological advances the new material feminisms represent namely breaking feminist waves (using Donna Haraway), cartography and its trans-disciplinarity (or 'postdisciplinarity').[3] These cannot be disentwined from the conceptual mediations they represent as part of the deep negotiation I have discussed regarding O'Brien's biosocial notion of reproduction.

---

1   Iris van der Tuin and Rick Dolphijn, 'The Transversality of New Materialism', *Women: A Cultural Review* 21:2 (2010): 153–71.

2   See Iris van der Tuin, 'Deflationary Logic: Response to Sara Ahmed's "Imaginary Prohibitions: Some Preliminary Remarks on the Founding Gesture of the 'New Materialism'"', *European Journal of Women's Studies* 15 (2008): 414–15.

3   Van der Tuin and Dolphijn, 'The Transversality of New Materialism'; Lykke, *Feminist Studies: A Guide to Intersectional Theory, Methodology, and Writing*, New York: Routledge, 2010.

Introducing the New Material Feminisms

In recent years there has been an emergence of interdisciplinary feminist theory that emphasizes materiality as part of a 'discontent with the social constructionist orthodoxy'.[4] These new material feminisms, variously referred to (for example 'the new materialism',[5] 'new feminist materialisms',[6] or simply 'material feminisms'[7]) renegotiate the biological essentialist and social constructionist binary, and constitute what has been called the material turn,[8] the ontological turn,[9] or the post constructionist turn.[10] This includes a number of vital, ground-breaking material feminist texts from across the disciplines such as Susan Hekman and Stacy Alaimo's *Material Feminisms*, Gillian Howie's *Between Feminism and Materialism*, and Michael Hames-Garcia and Paula Moya's *Reclaiming Identity*, as well as disability theorist Rosemarie Garland-Thomson in 'Misfits: A Feminist Materialist Disability Concept'.[11] These new texts analyse the effects of a once-radical feminist constructionism that has, arguably, become

---

4   Stacy Alaimo and Susan Hekman, eds, *Material Feminisms*, Bloomington: Indiana University Press, 2008, 90.

5   Sara Ahmed, 'Open Forum Imaginary Prohibitions: Some Preliminary Remarks on the Founding Gestures of the "New Materialism"', *European Journal of Women's Studies* 15:1 (2008): 23–39.

6   Iris van der Tuin, 'New Feminist Materialisms', *Women's Studies International Forum* 34 (2011): 271–7.

7   Alaimo and Hekman, *Material Feminisms*.

8   Ahmed, 'Open Forum Imaginary Prohibitions'; Myra J. Hird, 'Feminist Matters: New Materialist Considerations of Sexual Difference', *Feminist Theory* 5:2 (2004): 223–32.

9   Cecilia Asberg, 'Enter Cyborg: Tracing the Historiography and Ontological Turn of Feminist Technoscience Studies', *International Journal of Feminist Technoscience* 1:1 (2010); Maureen McNeil, 'Keynote presentation opening of the Posthumanities Hub', Linkoping University, 6 October 2009.

10   Cecilia Asberg and Nina Lykke, 'Feminist Technoscience Studies', *European Journal of Women's Studies* 17:4 (2010): 299–305.

11   For a few see Lynda Birke and Cecilia Asberg, 'Biology is a Feminist Issue: Interview with Lynda Birke', *European Journal of Women's Studies* 17:4 (2010): 413–23; Kath Woodward and Sophie Woodward, *Why Feminism Matters: Feminism Lost and Found*, Basingstoke: Palgrave Macmillan, 2009; Linda Martin Alcoff, 'Who's Afraid of Identity Politics?' in *Reclaiming Identity: Realist Theory and the Predicament of Postmodernism*, ed. Paula M.L. Moya and Michael R. Hames-Garcia, California: University of California Press, 2000, 312–44; Stevi Jackson, 'Why a Materialist Feminism is (Still) Possible – and Necessary', *Women's Studies International Forum* 24:3/4 (2001): 283–93; Noela Davis, 'New Materialism and Feminism's Anti-Biologism: A Response to Sara Ahmed', *European Journal of Women's Studies* 16:1 (2009): 67–80; Alexandra Howson, *Embodying Gender*, London: Sage Publishers, 2005; Diana Coole and Samantha Frost, eds, New *Materialisms: Ontology, Agency, and Politics*, Durham and London: Duke University Press, 2010; Karen Barad, *Meeting the Universe Halfway: Quantum Physics and the Entanglement of Matter and Meaning*, Durham and London: Duke University Press, 2007.

institutionally entrenched while acknowledging the continuity of thought from across the modern/postmodern spatio-temporal designation. For example, Nina Lykke believes that the new materialist feminisms, best described as 'post-constructionism', are indebted to feminist de/constructionism 'from Beauvoir to Butler' and that 'very few of the feminist theorists who argue for a rethinking of sex, biology, and embodiment would deny the genealogical kinship with feminist de/constructionism'.[12] Significantly, then, this re-engagement has the advantage of decades of feminist insight about the co-constitutive relationship between representation and reality regarding sex/gender and embodiment, a hallmark of postmodern thought though not exclusive to that approach.[13] Some key players in the linguistic turn are also important to the material turn, most notably Haraway, which demonstrates the emphasis on continuity of thought instead of discontinuity and breakage that I argue is a hallmark of this turn.

I will outline the new feminist materialisms as Lykke's post-constructionism but using the terms as interchangeable, but I favour post-constructionism as a new 'thinking technology' (borrowing Haraway's wording) that best describes its capacity to transcend the feminist constructionist/essentialist impasse because it breaks away from any (temporal and conceptual) limitations associated with the feminist waves model.

One familiar thread of the feminist waves narrative is a 'modern' second-wave of feminism as overtaken by a 'postmodern' third-wave. A major conceptual underpinning of generational feminist waves is a tension between 'essentialist' modern feminist epistemology and 'anti-essentialist' (or constructionist) postmodern epistemology presented as irreconcilable, and linked to feminism's 'anachronism' or 'death'. Many recent approaches convincingly undermine received knowledge that the modern – postmodern relationship is explained in a second to third wave antagonism, contending that such representations detract from feminism's actual complex diversity (over time, and at a time) the consequences of which are denial of conflicts or contestations, as the inevitable and even productive reality of wide-ranging, diverse situated knowledges playing out in Western feminist theory.[14]

---

12   Nina Lykke, 'The Timeliness of Post-Constructionism', *NORA – Nordic Journal of Feminist and Gender Research* 18:2 (June 2010): 132.

13   See for example, Ahmed, 'Open Forum Imaginary Prohibitions' and Lykke, 'The Timeliness of Post-Constructionism'.

14   See Van der Tuin, 'Deflationary Logic'; Clare Hemmings, 'Generational Dilemmas: A Response to Iris van der Tuin's "'Jumping Generations': On Second- and Third-Wave Feminist Epistemology'", *Australian Feminist Studies* 24:59 (2009): 33–7; Linda Alcoff and Gillian Howie, 'Breaking Feminist Waves', Series Foreword in *Between Feminism and Materialism: A Question of Method*, ed. Gillian Howie, New York: Palgrave Macmillan, 2010; Marysia Zalewski, *Feminism after Postmodernism: Theorising Through Practice*, London and New York: Routledge, 2000; Woodward and Woodward, *Why Feminism Matters*; Lykke, *Feminist Studies*.

Considering this rift in terms of Wendy Brown's 'wounded attachments' is a fitting caveat. Contemporary feminism remains challenged to construct political selves without becoming trapped into an oppositional self/other framework; Nietzsche's *ressentiment* or 'the moralizing revenge of the powerless'.[15] According to Brown identity politics and feminism, in particular, ends up reinforcing the very 'wounded attachments' it aims/claims to sever. The risk in identity politics based on recognition of patterns of historical subjugation of particular groups by others, is a dualistic political psychology that reproduces roles of victimhood and empowerment in ultimately reactionary and defeatist ways.[16]

These new material feminisms are associated with what Linda Alcoff and Howie refer to as a 'breaking feminist waves' methodology which circumvents the limitations of a linear progression to an end goal that is associated with the waves metaphor and counteracts reliance on the characterization of dualistic, unsettleable, and antagonistic differences in feminism, such as second versus third wave, and essentialist versus constructionist views of women's subject positions.[17] Post-constructionist, material feminist theories position themselves to take the best from the history of feminist theory without regard for the well-worn divide to address the 'material discursive' constitution of bodies and material life.[18] As Lykke aptly describes: 'The aim of these endeavours is to theorize bodily and trans-corporeal materialities in ways that neither push feminist thought back into the traps of biological determinism or cultural essentialism, nor make feminist theorizing leave bodily matter and biologies "behind" in a critically under-theorized limbo'.[19]

Feminism between Modernity and Postmodernity

In the sense that both postmodernism and feminism are critical of the androcentric 'underlying principles and beliefs of modernity' they share a political platform.[20] For example, radical feminism approaches postmodernism in its deconstruction of the Enlightenment underpinnings of patriarchy, including its discursive constructions

---

15   'Identity Politics', *Stanford Encyclopedia of Philosophy*, Stanford University, 2002.

16   See Woodward and Woodward, *Why Stories Matter*, which examines this complex dynamic/phenomenon in terms of a history of Western feminism and the narratives that are told there.

17   *Breaking Feminist Waves* is a series from Palgrave Macmillan, with a foreword written by Linda M. Alcoff and Gillian Howie.

18   Alaimo and Hekman, *Material Feminisms*.

19   Lykke, 'The Timeliness of Post-Constructionism', 131–2.

20   Jacquetta Newman and Linda A. White, *Women, Politics, and Public Policy: The Political Struggles of Canadian Women*, Don Mills, Ontario: Oxford University Press, 2006.

of 'women' (for instance in unattainable beauty standards and pornography).[21] At the same time, however, because postmodernism's cutting edge does not consider the modern roots of feminism off bounds, its radical deconstruction of the concept of 'woman' goes on to threaten the traditional foundation of movements for gender liberation. It is because of this complication that so much ink has been spilt coming to grips with what can be created by the merging of these two theoretically complex and internally diverse systems of thought.[22]

Postmodernity is not all 'post' or anti-modern, nor is feminism all modern. Feminism is not adequately defined as part of the modern project which postmodernism wishes to deconstruct, at least partly because it also sought to deconstruct Enlightenment modernity's values and traditions. Indeed, it did so before postmodernism.[23] The 'modern' notions of 'the subject' and 'the body' remain significant for feminist scholars, however, because they remain central for women in general. Some scholars, especially Dorothy Smith, have described feminism's particular orientation as being suspended between modernity and postmodernity, which implies a possible strategic use of the tools of both frameworks.[24] Like some forms of postmodernism, feminism is critical of patriarchy and provides tools for its dismantling, yet it is cautious about postmodernism's indiscriminate deconstructions that potentially culminate in a paralysing relativism, and its tendencies toward neo-determinism based on a socially over-determined body.[25]

The paralysing crux of the matter for feminists in the face of postmodernism's challenges, at least according to the conventional narrative, is that they cannot have it both ways – '[f]eminist theory cannot claim both that knowledge and the self are constituted within history and culture and that feminist theory speaks on behalf of a universalized "woman". Rather, it must embrace differences between women and accept a position of partial knowledge(s)'.[26] This presentation of the feminist dilemma tasks feminism with the impossible choice between its liberatory

---

21   Zalewski, *Feminism after Postmodernism*.

22   For example Linda Nicholson, ed., *Feminism/Postmodernism*, New York: Routledge, 1990; Zalewski, *Feminism after Postmodernism*; Newman and White, *Women, Politics, and Public Policy*.

23   Susan Bordo, 'Feminism, Foucault and the Politics of the Body', in *Up Against Foucault: Explorations of Some Tensions between Foucault and Feminism*, ed. Caroline Ramazanoglu, London: Routledge, 1993, 179–202; M.E. Bailey, 'Foucauldian Feminism: Contesting Bodies, Sexuality and Identity', in *Up Against Foucault*, ed. Caroline Ramazanoglu, 99–122; Somer Brodribb, *Nothing Mat(t)ers: A Feminist Critique of Postmodernism*, Toronto: James Lorimer and Company, 1993.

24   Dorothy Smith, 'Ironies of Post-Modernism or Cheal's Doom', *Canadian Journal of Sociology* 15:3 (1990): 334–45.

25   Alaimo and Hekman, *Material Feminisms*; Alcoff, 'Who's Afraid of Identity Politics?'.

26   Sue Thornham, 'Postmodernism and Feminism (or: Repairing our own cars)', in *The Routledge Critical Dictionary of Postmodern Thought*, ed. Stuart Sim, New York: Routledge, 1999, 41–52; See also Alison Stone, 'Essentialism and Anti-Essentialism in

(modern) roots and assumptions, and a (postmodern) critique of their patriarchal character. Lost in this never-ending loop, feminist agency is foreclosed; but is this the only way?

Third Wave Feminism and the 'Post-Natural' Body

Feminist theorists have risen to the challenge of reconceiving dualism in a variety of ways that validate the various and changeable experiences of women's embodiment by recognizing their experiences as different from each other, not just from men's. As Barbara Arneil claims that the defining feature of a 'third wave' of Anglo-Western feminism is a focus on differences among women, and differential embodiment.[27] Partly in response to the postmodern deconstruction of second wave feminist terms, especially as pertains to 'the body', in the late 1980s and early 1990s 'third wave' feminism emerged. Critiquing the universal woman and feminist activism's attachment to a naturalized body, third-wave feminists posit a body that embraces, to varying degrees, postmodern conceptions of the subject, power, and embodiment. The third wave 'body' attempts to break down Cartesian dualism through a more radical constructivism that renders 'natural' sex and 'cultural' gender inseparable. However, the third wave preoccupation with difference often translates into dismissal of the features of the modern body such as sex/gender, most featured in biological determinist arguments, and on which politically relevant commonalities among women are based.

Consequently, most third wave feminists posit versions of a 'post-natural body'; 'post-natural' in that it is not determined by its genes, nor its social mores, but by a more complex interaction between the two. Nature does not determine its features, nor does the social context – but the materiality of the body does fade in this analysis. Illustrating this disembodying tendency within feminism, Susan Stryker argues that the '"post-natural" body' is definitive of the third wave of feminism.[28] Stryker highlights the centrality of embodied difference to the newest feminisms, by focusing on the 'kind of difference represented by transsexuals', which she

---

Feminist Philosophy', *Journal of Moral Philosophy* 1:2 (2004) and Nicholson, *Feminism/ Postmodernism*.

27   What is captured in the term 'third-wave feminism' is hard to delineate. To some it is a tendency shared by several feminisms which seeks to transcend the second wave neglect of differences among women, which results from prioritizing differences between women and men. Its effects are not limited to those feminists who consider themselves part of the third wave rather than the second, however, since it destabilizes concepts held by both. I agree with Arneil that third wave feminism is best understood as an 'evolution in feminist thought generally, as it grapples towards particular, embodied, women's perspective(s)'; Barbara Arneil, *Politics and Feminism*, Oxford and Malden, MA: Wiley-Blackwell, 1999, 188.

28   Marysia Zalewski, 'A Conversation with Susan Stryker', *International Feminist Journal of Politics* 5:1 (March 2003): 122.

claims is 'a precursor to a whole range of issues around biomedical technology and the "post-natural" body'.[29] For example, the thorny gender categorizations raised by the issue of Androgen Insensitivity Syndrome (AIS) is particularly illuminating of the status of the 'natural' body in the third wave. AIS is a condition which prevents some genetically 'male' bodies from metabolizing testosterone, and thus from developing male genital structure. Second Wave feminist Germaine Greer's insistence on calling those with AIS 'men', her '"chromosomal fundamentalism", [and] a belief that X and Y chromosomes determine who is a man and who is a woman' leads to Stryker's observation that she 'seems not to recognize that the relationships between sexed embodiment, social role and psychological identity are very complex, and that there are more than two paths to gendered personhood'.[30]

Reconsidering Haraway

Feminist philosopher of science Haraway is at the intersection of the modern to postmodern turn. On the one hand, Newman and White are representative when they consider Haraway's famous 'A Cyborg Manifesto' (1985) as marking a paradigm shift in feminist practice from a focus on women as agential self-directed subjects of feminist politics, to querying women's subjectivity as constitutive of power that can be counterproductive to feminist aims. On the other hand, she is also sometimes considered the grandmother of the material turn as well. In spite of the difficulty in ideologically placing her, her work is indicative of the kind of respect of conceptual and methodological complexity required by the material turn in feminist theory. Furthermore, that Lykke claims Haraway as the central figure of feminist post-constructionism and Nancy Hartsock similarly considers Haraway an exemplary feminist standpoint theorist reinforces my point that she straddles, even bridges, seemingly divergent impulses and categories in the history of Western feminist thought.

Haraway rose to the challenge by presenting the concept of 'situated knowledges' which attempt to bridge the gulf between female sexed and reproductive bodies and women's multiple experiences of them. The difference between such theories and the old essentialism is in the idea of a new 'nomadic' subject described as 'the site of multiple, complex, and potentially contradictory sets of experiences, defined by overlapping variables such as class, race, age, lifestyle, sexual preference and others'.[31] The most obvious of these might be Haraway's famous and controversial cyborg figure which presents a version of complex feminist embodiment, however, it is her argument for a feminist objectivity constituted of partial position that is most significant.[32] It is here that her hopes to keep hold of both the objectivity

---

29 Zalewski, 'A Conversation with Susan Stryker', 121.
30 Zalewski, 'A Conversation with Susan Stryker', 118.
31 Zalewski, 'A Conversation with Susan Stryker', 121.
32 See Asberg, 'Enter Cyborg'; Lykke, *Feminist Studies*.

aspirations of feminism and the undeniable uncertainty of the traditional grounds of women's (common) experience are made clear. By contrast, while 'A Cyborg Manifesto' revolutionized feminist theory and practice, it also produced (like for Judith Butler) what she herself did not intend; it was taken up in such a way that it fed into the linguistic/constructionist turn in feminism with not altogether beneficial consequences for the movement as I will explore.[33]

The significance of Haraway's 'Situated Knowledges' is its direct attention to the dilemmas postmodernist theory posed to feminism in undoing the universal 'woman'. Haraway's answer to the constitutive dangers of false objectivity in feminist theory is that 'only partial perspective promises objective vision'. 'Feminist objectivity is about limited location and situated knowledge, not about transcendence and splitting of subject and object. It allows us to become answerable for what we learn how to see'.[34] Conceptually, she reconfigures sex/gender, or 'feminist critical empiricism versus radical constructionism' in recognition of the failure of bi-polar structures for any successful new feminist work. She critiques biological determinism (as a mark of postmodernist anti-essentialism) and yet writes, 'to lose authoritative biological accounts of sex, which set up productive tensions with gender, seems to be to lose too much; it seems to be to lose not just analytic power within a particular Western tradition but also the body itself as anything but a blank page for social inscriptions'.[35] Haraway's settlement is seeing the subjects as 'material-semiotic' actors, which holds both ends of the pole in view but still subverts the dualistic metaphor.[36] That is, it recognizes that a discursive understanding of the body emerges from the social experience of something named a body, the language becomes embodied.

Haraway's theorization of embodiment demonstrates her argument that the overlaps and intersections of nature and culture, human and machine, and animal and human, actually overlap and are never fixed or stable. The cyborg image stresses the intimacy between organism and machine as an 'integrated circuit', an information network unhindered by boundaries and specifically the dualisms of Western enlightenment narratives. Therefore, Haraway posits a post-human figure for feminists to embrace as a metaphor for the discursive material realities of being in a technological age. She tells us the 'self feminists must code' has changed into the cyborg, 'a kind of disassembled and reassembled personal self' not easily linked to a biological body.[37]

---

33   See Alaimo and Hekman, *Material Feminisms*, 86–7 and Asberg, 'Enter Cyborg', 19.

34   Donna Haraway, 'Situated Knowledges: The Science Question in Feminism and the Privilege of Partial Perspective', *Feminist Studies* 14:3 (1988): 593.

35   Haraway, 'Situated Knowledges', 591.

36   Haraway, 'Situated Knowledges', 593.

37   Donna Haraway, 'A Cyborg Manifesto: Science, Technology, and Socialist-Feminism in the Late Twentieth Century', in *Simians, Cyborgs, and Women: The Reinvention of Nature*, ed. Donna Haraway, New York: Routledge, 1991, 163.

Her work's significance here is its clear statement of desire to cross boundaries while maintaining a postmodern politics, even as it complicates the possibility for feminist identity. She explains: 'to recognize "oneself" as fully implicated in the world, frees us of the need to root politics in identification, vanguard parties, purity, and mothering'.[38] Women and cyborgs are hybrids, 'non-innocent monsters' implicated in the creation of new 'worlds' for better and worse. This is as much a statement about Haraway's postmodern conception of power as it is about the place of women within it.

In this way Lykke provides the best example of how to reclaim postmodernism, highlighting the limitations of such labels, particularly regarding Haraway.[39] In suggesting that Haraway's cyborg prefigured the material turn, Lykke argues that its hegemonic uptake in feminist studies 'is obscuring that the unfolding of synergies between feminist and post-modernist thought has taken a diversity of routes and sometimes gone beyond post-modernist anti-foundationalism'.[40] When feminist theorists succumb to the tendency to classify Haraway, and others like her, as simply postmodern anti-essentialists, they miss the category-thwarting nuances that post-constructionism takes as the starting point for new work.[41] Feminist materialism enables an understanding of why Haraway fits nowhere (or in multiple places at once), and a more realistic framework of categorization within feminist studies generally.

However, while it is easy to understand Haraway's motivation to replace patriarchal dichotomies so inadequate to the task of representing the complexity of women's existence, how this new space can support political agency involving embodied actors remains open ended as a matter of principle. Haraway's cyborg can be seen as merely one demonstration of such situated knowledges and partial perspectives, a point supported by her presentation of a number of other such figures (like the coyote, trickster, and oncomouse).[42] The cyborg then, was a historically specific, provocative tool for new thinking, but by undermining key dualisms it not only creatively resituates historically subjugated knowledges, but helps to effect the depoliticization and dis-integration of the material body and so, of the grounds for feminism. As Lynda Birke also recognized, since the emphasis is placed on the body's coextension with the rest of the world in an open network of information flow, its bounded internal features – its integrity, in a word – is what's lost. 'Information flows are all, and we thereby lose any sense of the organism itself'.[43]

Haraway echoes Butler's anti-essentialism in writing: 'There is nothing about being female that naturally binds women. There is not even such a state as "being"

---

38 Haraway, 'A Cyborg Manifesto', 1991, 176.

39 See also Asberg, 'Enter Cyborg'.

40 Lykke, *Feminist Studies*, 133.

41 Haraway, 'A Cyborg Manifesto', 2004, 19.

42 See Haraway, 'A Cyborg Manifesto', 2004, 19.

43 Lynda Birke, *Feminism and the Biological Body*, Edinburgh: Edinburgh University Press, 1999, 144.

female, itself a highly complex category constructed in contested sexual scientific discourses and other social practices'.[44] As Birke aptly argues, 'It is not only discourses ... that construct my boundaries, but also the various cells that are busily making and remaking my tissues'.[45]

All is not lost however, as Haraway's point in 'A Cyborg Manifesto' is outside the question of gender difference versus sex, that is, outside the binary metastructures of thought that are as damaging as unaccountable. To pick on details seems to lose the greater significance of her work's aptly recognized place in the history of feminist science studies. My point here is that Haraway's wish that cyborg feminism would be 'more able to remain attuned to specific historical and political positionings and permanent partialities *without abandoning the search for potent connections*' remains unfulfilled.[46] The recent proliferation of writing on the new material feminisms that are concerned with the feminist turn 'to discourse at the expense of the material' attests to this both explicitly and implicitly.[47] Nonetheless, Haraway remains on task in this turn. In *Material Feminisms*, Hekman and Alaimo credit her with keeping a grasp of matter without losing the analytical depth of social constructionism in discussing her concept of the '"material-discursive"', which refuses to separate the two'.[48]

'Breaking Feminist Waves'

This brings us back to the dualism of second wave versus third wave feminist theory that is associated with the metaphor of the waves. As I have previously signalled, one of the best contemporary feminist insights associated with the material turn entails the subversion of feminism's presentation as adequately captured in a waves analogy, especially as it positions modern, second wave feminisms in conflict with postmodern third wave feminisms.[49] Feminist theorists like Alcoff and Howie, Marysia Zalewski, Kath and Sophie Woodward mitigate feminism's representation as trapped between modernity and postmodernity by critiquing, and offering an alternative to, the waves metaphor. For example, Alcoff and Howie critique that such presentation sets up a chronological and teleological view of feminist theory that tends to work against positive frames for new work (among other deleterious effects).[50] Furthermore, I agree with Howie that:

---

44   Haraway, 'A Cyborg Manifesto', 1991, 155.
45   Birke, *Feminism and the Biological Body*, 144–5.
46   Haraway, 'A Cyborg Manifesto', 2004, 1. Emphasis added.
47   Hekman in Alaimo and Hekman, *Material Feminisms*, 86–7.
48   Alaimo and Hekman, *Material Feminisms*, 4.
49   Woodward and Woodward, *Why Feminism Matters*; Zalewski, *Feminism after Postmodernism*.
50   Gillian Howie, *Between Feminism and Materialism: A Question of Method*, New York: Palgrave Macmillan, 2010, vii.

'Dialogue between liberal feminists, radical, Marxist, and postmodernist feminists will enable us to organize around problems as they emerge and impact on diverse situations ...'.[51]

This new thinking about representing feminism will be an integral part of its renaissance because it makes possible attempts to fully access and reclaim diverse feminist theories without regard to entrenched disputes, whether characterized as generational or ideological. 'Breaking feminist waves' seems a natural outgrowth of difference feminism and diversity battles within feminism arising around the linguistic turn. In these new iterations it comes across that there is a coherence to the generational divisions, but that they shouldn't be misinterpreted as homogenous slices of history.[52] A further consequence of this approach emphasizes the ideological complexity of any wave of feminism making room for creative cross-generational (and cross-conceptual) combinations as Zalewski, and Woodward and Woodward exemplify.

Zalewski puts into engagement 'seemingly radically opposed' thinkers like Andrea Dworkin and Butler; while Woodward and Woodward make comparisons between the thinking of, for example, Luce Irigaray and Ariel Levy, and argue that Betty Friedan's centrally important book, *The Feminine Mystique,* had clear links with Irigaray and Cixous, even though they are rarely considered together because the former is seen as empirical, and the others as psychoanalytic.[53] As Woodward and Woodward aptly put it, 'Whilst it is always important to consider a writer in context, it is equally important not to be bound by dualities of discipline or academic traditions'.[54]

While such combinations may not be unique to new material feminisms, that they are emerging as part of a larger trans-dualistic, 'postdisciplinary' framework is. Lykke explains a postdisciplinary, or postdiscipline, discipline implies an area regarded as '*both* as an independent field of knowledge production (with its own core-object, theories, reflections on methodologies, epistemologies and ethics) *and* as a transgressive field that, through its multi-, inter-, trans- and postdisciplinary practices, engages in radically open transversal dialogue across and beyond traditional disciplinary boundaries'.[55] At the same time, breaking feminist waves, also enables a robust and mature focus on commonalities.

Another important way the cross-feminist waves way of looking at ideas and feminist practices holds possibility for a renewed feminism is the recognition of not just differences among women in a spatio-temporal sense, but also similarities.

---

51   Howie, *Between Feminism and Materialism*, 205.

52   See Alcoff and Howie in Howie, *Between Feminism and Materialism*; Woodward and Woodward, *Why Feminism Matters*; and Zalewski, *Feminism after Postmodernism*.

53   See also work on Simone de Beauvoir in, for example, Woodward and Woodward, *Why Feminism Matters* and Sonia Kruks, 'Simone de Beauvoir: Engaging Discrepant Materialisms', in Coole and Frost, *New Materialisms*, 259.

54   Woodward and Woodward, *Why Feminism Matters*, 168.

55   Lykke, *Feminist Studies*, 209–10.

Howie puts this best by deeply reconsidering and rearticulating the notion that internationalism must present a stumbling block to feminism. She resituates feminism writing: 'The recognition that dwelling exceeds spatial relations, that place is a function of the social imaginary constituted through competing interests, and that the particular is fastened within a global network of relations, alliances, and movements provides momentum to coalitional feminism'.[56] The intersectionality of space and time is fore-grounded because 'the relationship between the local and the global is not to be defined in terms of geography or territory but as existing simultaneously and mutually constitutive'.[57] Howie's argument for a feminist re-visitation of materialism culminates in the conclusion that to answer the old structure and agency debate, *either/or* frameworks will not do.

Key among the theorists constituting the new methodological paradigm is Zalewski in *Feminism after Postmodernism* which systematically investigates the 'alleged gulf' between modernist and postmodernist feminisms, both theoretically and by applying each purported approach to dilemmas surrounding new reproductive technologies.[58] Her purpose is practical; to mediate between and address the presentation of more traditional feminisms as anachronistic and feminism's quietude over the last few decades because of its imbrication in the essentialist/constructionist loggerhead. She effectively illustrates the convergences as well as the divergences of the radical, liberal, and Marxist (modernist) feminisms with the psychoanalytic (postmodernist) ones – which breaks down the hardened view of two opposing, chronological camps. Her approach also demonstrates how attending to particular material issues, like reproduction, can help revive feminist activism. The subtle message is that these radically opposed differences are theoretically articulated and enacted, but in practice they lose (much) of their significance.

Most significantly and like Howie, Zalewski clarifies that neither modernist nor postmodernist feminisms are accurately nor usefully explained in this absolutist *either/or* framework. That is, feminism is neither modern nor postmodern, but in reality encompasses a range of approaches between two extremes. Furthermore, this placement is creative, and productive in keeping with the analogy. She writes,

> There is a profound ambiguity in feminism: it challenges modernist epistemology but is located in the emancipatory impulses of modernism. So in a sense *all* feminisms are in an anomalous position vis-à-vis the modernist/postmodernist debate. The idea of a gulf seems inadequate to capture this intriguing ambiguity. Instead it encourages a policing and disciplining set of strategies.[59]

---

56   Howie, *Between Feminism and Materialism*, 203.
57   Howie, *Between Feminism and Materialism*.
58   Zalewski, *Feminism after Postmodernism*.
59   Zalewski, *Feminism after Postmodern*, 141.

Negative and Positive Difference, or Beyond Dialectics?

Lykke's sophisticated theorization of the new material feminisms as post-constructionism similarly subverts linear temporality and its controversial conceptual implications, most clearly in refusing the prefix 'new'. She explains: 'Constructionist and post-constructionist feminist ways of theorizing are, as I see it, running in parallel'.[60] Ultimately, Lykke's 'post-constructionism' indicates continuities and discontinuities with de/constructionist feminisms that prevents simplified and misleading characterizations. Highlighting how post-constructionism is not a simple turning away from previous theory but a positive and progressive negotiation, she also emphasizes its central feature as 'the double move of going into and beyond post-modern epistemological thought and constructionist understandings of science ... rather than "sticking to Harding's more simple taxonomy, "post-modern feminist epistemology"'.[61] Lykke's neologisms are part of a more extensive lexicon of umbrella terms which highlights the temporary, unstable (always becoming or in process) character of the feminist epistemological and methodological frameworks she theorizes, and also their foundation in eclectic, or hybrid, theoretical traditions. Such a move is no mean feat – keeping diversity in focus, while facilitating dialogue and also avoiding the more controversial connotations of 'new' linked to 'sequential negation and progress narrative' as Van der Tuin and Dolphijn put it.[62]

On the other hand, Diana Coole and Samantha Frost clarify that such classification of emerging materialisms does not imply a denial of 'their rich materialist heritage'; instead 'their interventions might be categorized as *renewed* materialisms'.[63] Moreover, a vast and diverse collection of thinkers belongs under this banner, and especially the neo-Marxists or 'non-dogmatic (for example autonomist) Marxism'.[64] They refer to new materialisms to emphasize that the matter that is being theorized is 'unprecedented'. The world that Marx theorized did not entail the sort of technologies of production and reproduction that ours does even if he understood that environmental destruction may have been a part of it. But the unprecedented character of the new material feminisms for these authors also references that these diverse materialisms are also 'new paradigms for which no overall orthodoxy has yet been established'.

A final sense in which they are new is that this material/ontological turn understands its object of analysis, the material, as becoming rather than something that precedes human life activity (in its complex natural-sociality) but is itself an agent in that life/process. A similar denial of dualistic separation, before the

---

60   Lykke, *Feminist Studies*, 133.

61   Lykke, *Feminist Studies*, 133 and 134 respectively.

62   Lykke, *Feminist Studies*, 140; See also Van der Tuin and Dolphijn, 'The Transversality of New Materialism'.

63   Coole and Frost, *New Materialisms*, 4.

64   Coole and Frost, *New Materialisms*, 4 and 28 respectively.

fact, as it were – especially in light of material lived experience, for example in Barad's 'intra-action' which sees difference as enacted everywhere, all of the time through each engagement with the environment. This concept highlights the inter-relational constitution of subject and object or 'the intra-action of the observer, the observed and observing instruments, all of which are "agential"'.[65] Starting from quantum physics where unstable referents are changed by their encounters, Barad captures how this applies in the social world. The point is that reality is not observer-independent; reality is not 'built by things-in-themselves or things-behind-phenomena, but of things-in-phenomena'.[66] These neologisms and others like them capture the sort of theories constituting the post-constructionist turn, indicating the same trans-dualist emphasis in differing fields of analysis. They also indicate the emergence of a somewhat uniform, radical notion of difference as ubiquitous and constant, with material connotation as part of the one-in-the-sameness of being in knowing indicated by Barad's interrelated concept of onto-epistemology as discussed.

When matter is seen as agented, as in post-constructionist feminisms, it becomes possible to interact with matter in a way that affects both sides, and what is classified as 'matter' is opened up to include almost anything. As imbricated in the body/mind dichotomy, matter has been presented as negative differential. Dichotomies, in general, build on exclusion so always build on 'negative differentials' as in Hegelian dialectics and Derrida's system of signifiers, on which postmodern theory and discourse analysis usually build – to perpetuate categorization and division. But as Clare Colebrook exemplifies, one new materialist strategy is to change negative differentiating towards a 'positive difference'.[67] In this view difference is not negative (to be avoided and remedied) but seen as everywhere – all of the time – which allows differences to be seen as active processes. Lived embodiment is a process of movement and change, simultaneously entailing freedom and possibility, restraint and limit.

The fundamental point of difference of the new material feminisms however, is this break-through of the essentialist/constructionist binary. 'It is entirely possible ... to accept social constructionist arguments while also insisting that the material realm is irreducible to culture or discourse and that cultural artefacts are not arbitrary vis-à-vis nature'.[68] This trans-dualism has fundamental consequences that can't really be overstated. The feminist debate over whether recent materialist theories are justifiably described as 'new' reveals the need for a new view of spatial and temporal relations in feminist studies which is evident in the 'breaking

---

65   Van der Tuin and Dolphijn, 'The Transversality of New Materialism', 165.

66   Karen Barad cited in Matz Hammarstrom, 'On the Concepts of Transaction and Intra-action', *The Third Nordic Pragmatism Conference*, Uppsala, 1–2 June 2010, pp. 9–10. Conference paper.

67   Claire Colebrook, 'On Not Becoming Man: The Materialist Politics of Unactualized Potential', in Hekman and Alaimo, *Material Feminism*, 73–5.

68   Coole and Frost, *New Materialisms*, 27.

feminist waves' methodology emerging from such post-constructionist theories associated with cartography.

New materialism does not just expand or widen older kinds. It announces a fresh, transversal, but also meta-disciplinary methodology in feminist studies but much more broad in application. Though new materialism does represent the addition of 'bodily materiality *to* the economic' – this limited understanding misses the greater offering.[69] It is not simply 'new' in the teleological sense here (as others have noted) because earlier forms were more complex than recognized in academic renderings nor are they simply about conceptual advances, implied for example in the tradition of Hegelian dialectics (such as post positivist epistemologies as advancing upon positivist epistemologies).[70] Van der Tuin and Dolphijn explain, '[d]ue to the fact that causally linear reasoning has been left behind, it cannot be argued that new materialism entails a simple move *beyond* social constructionism in a progressive way'.[71] In resonance with Lykke's central argument about post-constructionism as a move into and beyond postmodern ideas, new materialisms are trans-dual in the sense of challenging linear teleology as ways of seeing – the most radical sense of theory – which has overlapping and intertwined spatial and temporal dimensions. Taken to one extreme, they call for new ways of portraying conceptual relationships to emphasize time/space intersections rather than clear cut and homogeneous lineage.

I have argued that the post-constructionist new material feminisms represent a 'breaking feminist waves' methodology because they challenge dualistic categorization (such as modern versus postmodern and second versus third wave feminism) which have significant spatial and temporal connotations. It is this linear and teleological model which underlies both senses of dualistic classification and which Van der Tuin and Dolphijn further break away from in theorizing the new material feminism's trans-dualist, or in their terms, 'transversal' methodology as cartography.

As I have explored, since the new material feminisms draw on old and new work and from across academic disciplines, they are translinear in a historical/temporal and spatial/conceptual sense, hence defy simply classification. This is why Van der Tuin and Dolphijn claim that, 'New materialism, then, takes scholarship into an absolute deterritorialisation and is not an epistemic class that has a clear referent'.[72] In place of linear temporality, they use 'Cartography rather than classification';[73] mapping rather than linear plotting on a time scale. It is a trans-linear approach mapping coimplications, for example as Lykke

---

69 Coole and Frost, *New Materialisms*, 160.

70 Coole and Frost, 161. See also for example, Lykke, 'The Timeliness of Post-constructionism', and Alcoff and Howie, 'Preface' in Howie, *Between Feminism and Materialism*.

71 Van der Tuin and Dolphijn, 'The Transversality of New Materialism', 157.

72 Van der Tuin and Dolphijn, 'The Transversality of New Materialism', 161.

73 Van der Tuin and Dolphijn, 'The Transversality of New Materialism', 166.

highlights, 'to stress how different positions in feminist epistemology have different methodological and ethical implications' that are intra-active, not one in the same or in progressive and linear in relation.[74] The cartographical method also includes as an essential feature, trans-disciplinarity.

Building from the 'Breaking Feminist Waves' point, the difficulties inherent in rigid characterization of the new material feminisms is largely down to classificatory paradigms which fail the conceptual terrain that is being charted. It's easy to get it wrong because modern epistemology defaults to disciplinary boundaries which these new materialisms are most accurately understood outside of.[75] 'New materialism criticizes not only the use of "a discipline" or "a paradigm" as pre-determined, but is critical also, along the lines of the dismantling of binary oppositions that it enacts, of the pre-determination of classifications of theoretical trends'.[76] We can think of this as Barad's intra-action at the institutional level. The new material feminisms are fundamentally trans-disciplinary; as phenomena they enact a 'disciplinary transversality'.[77] This has implications for the broader applications and reach of its methodological and conceptual (re)negotiations beyond feminist theory and toward a paradigm shift in contemporary cultural theory.[78] A significant stumbling block has been disciplinary boundaries or 'disciplinary territoriality' which distorts and reduces the actual scope and application of the new materialisms.[79] For example, it is because the trans-dual conceptual advances are beyond disciples in significance that they affect a deterritorializion. Because we as a rule, see the world, from our distinct disciplinary lenses (sociology or biology for example) we are already biased in our readings of new materialism something they call 'buying into disciplinary territoriality'.[80]

The gains for scholarly work, and conceptual understandings through which we come to understand and (mis)represent the world, in terms of dualism at present, are equally unbounded. This is a high stakes turn by which we stand to gain a lot within feminist theory, as we saw with the breaking feminist waves approach, but potentially much more than that.[81] Van der Tuin and Dolphijn in particular, elaborate and stretch the benefits in time and scope – backward into history (and forward, in theory), and meta-disciplinarily to scholarship more generally, including a sweep of thinkers who have been relegated to the sidelines because of academic trends of dualism. 'Modernist scholars like Bergson, Alfred

---

74   Lykke, *Feminist Studies*, 145.
75   Van der Tuin and Dolphijn, 'The Transversality of New Materialism', 159.
76   Van der Tuin and Dolphijn, 'The Transversality of New Materialism', 167.
77   Van der Tuin and Dolphijn, 'The Transversality of New Materialism', 162.
78   Van der Tuin and Dolphijn, 'The Transversality of New Materialism', 163.
79   Van der Tuin and Dolphijn, 'The Transversality of New Materialism', 161.
80   Van der Tuin and Dolphijn, 'The Transversality of New Materialism', 161.
81   See Birke and Asberg, 'Biology is a Feminist Issue'; Hekman in Alaimo and Hekman, *Material Feminisms*; and Van der Tuin and Dolphijn, 'The Transversality of New Materialism', 167.

North Whitehead, William James and Edmund Husserl', are among those great minds named as having 'been pushed aside or reinterpreted by dualist thinking'.[82]

More modestly, the 'transversality of new materialism' enables gains in feminist theory by reconsidering and re-evaluating the work of feminist theorists (including complex ideas that are not easily captured and/or readily invoke polarization, so are easily mischaracterized) from previous historical moments and traditions like that of O'Brien.[83] It goes back to hermeneutics for example when considering the widely varying interpretations of Donna Haraway, O'Brien, Butler, and even Hartsock, which are subject to, among many other things, changing academic trends.

The new material feminisms address the loss of matter's agency in both modern and postmodern accounts of embodiment and reproduction with the social overdeterminism of the biological. Van der Tuin and Dolphijn write, 'The strength of new materialism is precisely to be found in its ability to show that agential, or the *non-innocent* nature of all matter, seems to have escaped *both* modernist (positivist) and postmodernist humanist epistemologies'.[84] The point of difference between new material feminisms and previous approaches is that matter has agency. It is not simply (as) represented in scientific or sociological/cultural theory alike. They explain: 'whereas a modernist scientific materialism allows for one True representation of matter, and a postmodernist cultural constructivism allows for a plethora of equally true representations, it is the shared *representationalism* that is questioned and shifted by new materialism'.[85] This is in line with the equivocal feminist position vis-à-vis the resistance and embracing responses to NRTs, though in slightly different terms. There – matter – or reproductive materiality (for women in particular) is not deterministic, but a changing historical and biosocial process aided by policies and social practices that can help or hinder meaningful choice.

Conclusion

In essence, the new materialists argue that bodies are material; that is, products of complex biosocial processes which are neither simply nor primarily a biological fact, nor are they purely socially constructed artefacts. Meanings are attributed to bodies, and bodies come to reflect those meanings. That the meaning of biology is politically and culturally mediated is a cornerstone feminist insight richly and variously explained by scholars in the interdisciplinary field of feminist

---

82   Van der Tuin and Dolphijn, 'The Transversality of New Materialism', 167.

83   As has been the case with new scholarship on de Beauvoir, and Shulamith Firestone.

84   Van der Tuin and Dolphijn, 'The Transversality of New Materialism', 159.

85   Van der Tuin and Dolphijn, 'The Transversality of New Materialism', 164.

(techno)science studies since the 1970s.[86] But we know from at least as early as Wollstonecraft's *A Vindication of the Rights of Woman* that biological bodies are cultural and historical entities in process. However, the sort of rigid biology/ society binary that has been a significant feature of feminist discourse until now has limited an adequate or realistic understanding of women's lives. Anne Phillips states: 'the variety of women's interests does not refute the claim that interests are gendered. That some women do not bear children does not make pregnancy a gender neutral event'[87] and as I would suggest, seeing sex/gender as socially constructed does not mean that it is not also biological. Furthermore, because of women's rightly apprehensive engagement with all things biological because of their historic association with 'nature', feminism's actual engagement with the biological body outside of a reductive Cartesian framework has been limited.[88] But without refocusing on material rather than abstract forms of embodiment, feminism will remain at an ultimately unproductive (biological) essentialist versus (social) constructionist impasse at the foundation of the most difficult feminist issues especially regarding reproduction and new reproductive technologies.

In many significant respects the new material feminisms represent the most promising feminist approach to the constructionist/essentialist impasse especially as it plays out regarding NRTs. Biology, understood as historical and cultural process *and* materially grounded, can be reclaimed for feminism. In spite of biological determinism built on a false belief in natural bodies as passive matter, feminist biologist Lynda Birke aptly argues that 'biological knowledge can be a feminist ally'.[89] In specific, as diverse and emergent theories which insist on the interpenetration of biological and social realms, in various terminology, they constitute a methodological approach that has the greater consequence of 'breaking feminist waves'. As such they pose a broader challenge to oppositional narratives in terms of feminist theory (for example, second versus third wave feminism) or more general theoretical trends (modernist versus postmodernist). As discussed, such presentations signify dual and antagonistic conceptual, not only temporal, dimensions as well.

This allows an incorporation of the diversity of women's individual embodied sex/gender experiences, while still accounting for the corporeal commonalities women share. They also reignite recurring debates about feminism's and practical differences. In particular they are a potentially fruitful ground for the working out of the biosocial dialectic within feminism, and specifically in feminist technoscience studies, but also more broadly between divisions like the natural sciences and social sciences. Van der Tuin and Dolphijn, in particular, reveal how

---

86 For an excellent historiography of feminist technoscience studies see Asberg, 'Enter Cyborg'.

87 Anne Phillips, *The Politics of Presence*, Oxford: Clarendon Press, 1995, 68.

88 Birke and Asberg, 'Biology is a Feminist Issue', 414.

89 Birke and Asberg, 'Biology is a Feminist Issue', 415.

the trans-dualism or 'transversalism' of the new materialisms will have resonance far beyond feminist studies.

Contradictions are a necessary part of learning, of history and the momentum of embodied life itself, and shouldn't be interpreted as evidence of feminism's fracture into incommensurable ideological factions hence its final undoing. It is important not to shy away from theorists who undo tidy categories of analysis; in fact, this is what's needed to update and advance feminist thinking. Most simply, 'feminism [is] not a rulebook but a discussion, a conversation, a process'[90] – but one that must take into account even prioritize gendered embodiment along the lines of the hegemonic bifurcation of male and female and its onto-epistemological significance.

90   Tavi Gevenson, 'Still Figuring it Out', TedxTeen Talk, 31 March 2012.

Conclusion

In this book, I have been driven by the desire to understand women's paradoxical experiences of their reproductive bodies as ones of both vulnerability and power in patriarchal cultures. Key to unravelling this paradox is a history of birth appropriation underpinned by an androcentric dualism that continues to inform much sociopolitical and legal ideology and practice in liberal societies. I develop the claim that new reproductive technologies, which disembody female reproductive process, represent a new manifestation of an old paradigm of birth appropriation, which is deeply entrenched in Western politics and culture, especially those associated with postmodernism. I revisit Mary O'Brien's dialectical reproductive materialism, especially her view of the reproductive body as biosocial to elaborate the intertwined material, ideological and social significance of this change. On the conceptual level this entails a rather complicated proposition since O'Brien's work has been relegated to the sidelines of feminist theory in many respects that I explore as rooted in a tenacious and distorting mind/body, social constructionist/biological essentialist dualism that needs challenging in both mainstream and feminist political praxis though my focus here is on the latter and especially as it comes to bear on reproductive politics in Anglo-feminism from roughly 1980 to present day. My theorization of NRTs is a thoroughly material and dialectical understanding of reproduction as a biosocial process as situated in a rich and diverse history of feminist studies concerned with material embodiment that does not neglect biology. This renegotiation of nature and culture is mirrored in a number of excellent more recent works, especially those categorized as new material feminisms. In particular, Shiloh Whitney's concept of corporeality, and Garland Thomson's materialist concept of misfits demonstrate the culmination of feminist thinking about biosocial embodiment from a practical and philosophical standpoint.

At the heart of the paradox I have theorized is the deep-seated association of corporeality (and especially women's reproduction) with vulnerability taken in opposition to power. Even in the age of new reproductive technology (NRT) reproduction (pregnancy and birth) is a powerful reminder of the material origins of human life, but not often in its true complexity which is at least partly because they are experiences apprehended second hand from men who have constituted the hegemonic 'truth' of liberal individualism in Western society. In such presentations women's bodies, hence women, are predominantly portrayed in terms of vulnerability (and occasional veneration) rather than the actual paradoxical continuum of vulnerability and power they entail. Such misconstruals betray a greater struggle with the reality of human (inter) dependency since (as embodied agents) we all inevitably, and without exception, are dependent at various points throughout the life course; for instance when we are infants, ill, elderly and dying. This is often expressed in the history of political thought as the disenfranchisement of women, and others, whose deviation from the disembodied, rational (male) ideal come to symbolize bodily 'weaknesses' – dependence as opposed to independence – in an impossible (yet normatively entrenched) dualistic and oppositional framework.

O'Brien identified two 'moments' of 'world historic' significance; the discovery of physiological paternity, and the advent of mass contraceptive technology, because each altered human understandings of their relationship to nature, with paradoxical consequences especially for women. I have argued in this book that new reproductive technologies are a third such moment because they alter women's reproductive consciousness by separating sex and reproduction, and reproduction and parenthood. This shift is a 'masculinization' of women's reproduction because only men naturally experience sex as separate from reproduction, and reproduction as separate from parenthood. This change is of great significance because she, and I, consider reproduction in its dialectically entwined social, material and psychological dimensions. Moreover, NRTs contribute to a history of birth appropriation by disembodying women's reproductive processes, recreating them in the laboratory. For example, in vitro fertilization happens outside the human female body, rendering discrete and manipulable previously integrated aspects of reproduction. This cannot but have radical implications for women's reproductive experiences and associated epistemologies (for better or worse.)

Unpacking such a feminist argument involves appreciation of feminist social epistemologies as constituting a 'critique of the individualism of modern epistemology, and their corresponding reconstructions of epistemic subjects as *situated* knowers'.[1] I have discussed Karen Barad's concept of 'onto-epistemology', a complex theory blending quantum physics and feminist theory, and building on the belief that being and knowing are inseparable which entails an ethical dimension: 'Once feminists draw attention to the fact that knowing is something that we do and do through engagement with others, the ethical dimensions of knowing becomes apparent'.[2]

Ideas have history just as '[e]xistence is not an individual affair'.[3] We think in complex multilogue amongst others, both over time and at a time, as the postconstructionist shift from linear classification to cartography indicates. Linear classifications, such as timelines, suggest dualistic comparisons between

---

1   'Feminist Social Epistemology', Stanford Encyclopedia of Philosophy, Stanford University, 2006. Web. http://plato.stanford.edu/entries/feminist-social-epistemology/

2   Barad, 1998, footnote, 21. See also Nina Lykke. *Feminist Studies: A Guide to Intersectional Theory, Methodology, and Writing.* New York: Routledge, 2010, 141. 'Feminist Social Epistemology', 20.

3   Karen Barad. *Meeting the Universe Halfway: Quantum Physics and the Entanglement of Matter and Meaning.* USA: Duke University Press, 2007. i.

what comes before and after, while cartography or mapping is given to more transdual, multifactorial conceptualization. More specifically, feminist theories are inevitably informed by, and inform, more mainstream political theory including birth appropriation, underpinned by patriarchal dualism in political theory, which has played out in feminist debates, most importantly as oppositional positionings of biological essentialism and social constructionism. It also offers the opportunity for creative negotiations. I explore equivocal feminist responses to NRTs (Chapter 3) as the kind of significant mitigation of extreme positions (Chapter 2) that is conceptually mirrored in O'Brien's biosocial theory (Chapter 4), and feminist postconstructionist theories more generally (Chapter 5). Here Shiloh Whitney's attendance to the 'corporeality of vulnerability'[4] reveals the potential richness of encounters between orthodox and feminist political theory related to the body. Building from Eva Feder Kittay's feminist critique of 'normative independence' in liberal theories of personhood she demonstrates a way out of the power versus vulnerability dichotomy which is an extension of the biology versus society pairing that I have explored regarding reproduction.

To borrow Whitney's phrasing 'the facts of corporeal vulnerability' historically associated with women's reproductive capacity (as a recurring theme in canonical Western political theory, even relatively progressive ones such as Hobbes') are wrongly seen as biologically determined, hence unchangeable. Such misconstrual is damaging for women, in obvious ways, but moreover serves to perpetuate false dichotomies (like mind/body) and hegemonic individualism, which run counter to a fully human/situated embodiment (for example, being in love, or in lust, pregnant, or empathetic). Finally, the most meaningful and happy aspects of human life often lie in our interdependence with others; as Whitney writes, 'one of the things we affirm about personhood is the opportunity to care and be cared for'.[5] Most importantly, some of us will become pregnant and give birth which, paradoxically can be profoundly humanizing as well as fundamentally disintegrating on an individual level, and often both. In any case, women are in a particularly good position to counter this significantly distorting androcentric bias in Western politics and society as those who birth and still perform the majority of the care and nurturance of the vulnerable (children, the elderly, and sick) and, as a result, are unjustifiably disadvantaged in myriad ways.[6] Understanding new reproductive technologies as disembodying reproduction in light of a history of political ideas (which are entrenched in patriarchal dualism) adds gravity and urgency to studying NRTs. They become not simply neutral tools for changing social and political

---

4   Shiloh Whitney. 'Dependency Relations: Corporeal Vulnerability and Norms of Personhood in Hobbes and Kittay' *Hypatia* 26:3 (Summer 2011).

5   Whitney, 'Dependency Relations', 560.

6   Marilyn Waring. *Counting for Nothing: What Men Value and What Women are Worth.* Toronto: University of Toronto Press, 1999; Laura M. Purdy, 'What Can Progress in Reproductive Technology Mean for Women?' *The Journal of Medicine and Philosophy,* 21: 5 (1996): 507.

values, but also artefacts of a history of social struggle over bodily differences as linked to social norms with inequitable material consequences.

Whitney's reworking of Kittay and Hobbes' notions of personhood vis-à-vis dependency and autonomy theories, advances both by mediating vulnerability and power considered as mutually exclusive. Since Hobbes finds power in fleeing inherent human vulnerability (in social and political life) and pre-emptively rendering others vulnerable, and Kittay valorizes dependency relations associated with (vulnerable) women over independence associated with men, Whitney argues both theories reinforce the dichotomy of independence and dependence.[7] This is especially problematic for Kittay because it frustrates her aim to more fundamentally revalue dependency. Because the notion of vulnerability she examines is defined dichotomously it is 'in tension with its *corporeality* ... the turn to considering the person as an embodied life', which 'allow[s] for a more profound valorization of vulnerability'.[8] Whitney instead calls for a fundamentally resituated and wholly integrated understanding of corporeal vulnerability (or biology in Western thought more generally, including traditional understandings of reproduction) that are more in line with the contradictory social and material experiences we have of our bodies, as source of (often frustrating) fluctuation between dependence and independence. In Whitney's use of the term corporeality to mean the synthesis of the vulnerability and power dichotomy upheld and reproduced in political theory including feminist presentations of the body's greater significance it resonates with the embodiment I advocate.

In reinterpreting Kittay's *Love's Labor,* Whitney provides access to its more radical implications outside of a dualistic, 'wounded attachment' in Wendy Brown's terms. She argues that there are powers consistent with vulnerability, which helps explain the kind of paradoxical power that women's reproduction presents.[9] As I explored briefly in Chapter 1, and Whitney presents, Gail Weiss's research is exemplary in this regard because, flouting oppositional thinking 'her notion of bodily integrity is informed by and cultivated in the experiences of fluidity, permeability, incorporation, and transmogrification during pregnancy and other experiences of extensive bodily change'.[10] Such presentations are representative of

---

7   Whitney, 'Dependency Relations', 562. Also see 573, footnote 18.

8   Whitney, 'Dependency Relations', 570.

9   For example Whitney refers to 'motility and sensation' as 'not best understood as powers a body can have on its own, sovereign or autonomous powers opposed to vulnerability. They are instead relational, adaptive powers, dependent on a multitude of influences, balanced on multiple points of reference and resistance. Crucially, this means *they are powers that are consistent with vulnerability,* even complicit with vulnerability: powers whose development is inseparable from the adaptation and cultivation of specific vulnerabilities', 'Dependency Relations', 570.

10   Whitney, 'Dependency Relations', 570. See also, for example, Imogen Tyler's work.

feminist standpoint epistemology in that they normalize women's (reproductive) subject positions and directly subvert the (androcentric) liberal individual (literally 'one who cannot be divided') on which Western citizenship is founded. As Whitney refreshingly points out, 'a more inclusive affirmation of personhood [is] one that does not choose between independence and dependence, but reconceives them both in light of the visceral particularities of human relationality'.[11] This allows us to understand independence in its true context of an embodied life (including birth, development, illness, aging, and death) which highlights dependency's perennial rather than exceptional character, and moreover, its value.[12] This was what O'Brien also argued for in theorizing reproduction as a material process that incorporated inseparably historical and biological features, which are experienced personally, if also collectively, in specific social and temporal instances. Most importantly, and as many feminist care ethicists have also argued, not only is embodiment not to be denied and avoided, but it must be valued – something which calls for reorientation to seeing lived embodiment as a process, at any given moment but also over time, for example by '[f]ocusing on vulnerabilities in the context of the whole life ...'.[13]

The repositioning of the concept of vulnerability in the context of an embodied life course links Whitney to disability theorist, Garland-Thomson's proposal of misfit as 'a feminist materialist disability concept'. For the latter, '[v]ulnerability is a way to describe the potential for misfitting to which all human beings are subject'.[14] Misfitting, more commonly associated with disability, for Garland-Thomson is a universal condition that is sometimes latent as a function of its context-specific character.[15] We are disabled only when we misfit with the world which is something that happens to all of us as a condition of relation or encounter, and this moves the 'idea of dissonance from epistemology into phenomenology'.[16]

The phenomena of fitting or misfitting with the world, places the experience of vulnerability in the material situation, the spatiotemporal location of the event. Fitting or misfitting is a happening, rather than a fixed characteristic of the body. Whether one fits or misfits in any given moment, changes and is contingent on the fluid process of bodies over a life course intra-acting with an equally constantly changeable material environment. She clearly states: 'A misfit occurs when world fails flesh in the environment one encounters – whether it is a flight of stairs, a boardroom full of misogynists, an illness or injury, a whites-only country club, sub-zero temperatures, or a natural disaster'.[17]

---

11   Whitney, 'Dependency Relations', 570.
12   Whitney, 'Dependency Relations', 569.
13   Whitney, 'Dependency Relations', 569.
14   Rosemarie Garland-Thomson, 'Misfits: A Feminist Materialist Disability Concept', *Hypatia* 26:3 (Summer, 2011): 593.
15   Garland-Thomson, 'Misfits', 600.
16   Garland-Thomson, 'Misfits', 601.
17   Garland-Thomson, 'Misfits', 593, 600.

Misfitting applies particularly well to women as reproductive misfits in patriarchal cultures in spite of the androcentric NRTs which offer women the chance to reproduce like men. I would add that a misfit occurs when, as Charlotte Witt has exemplified, a pregnant woman in 1946 is denied access to graduate school because Harvard University did not admit pregnant women, and a mother in 1939 quits her job because the norms of maternity in that place and time 'precluded women from working outside the home'.[18] In an ongoing sense, women's reproduction creates ethico-onto-epistemological discord when, for example, would-be mothers (academic and otherwise) forego childbirth altogether because of the particular misfits of professional and corporeal lives.

To be disabled is *to* 'misfit' and to *be a* misfit, outside the invisible norms of personhood and also to know the world from a position of subjugated knowledge from which a 'politicized identity might arise'.[19] This hearkens back to Hartsock's feminist standpoint theory as rooted in the political consciousness of differing, hierarchically ordered social positions with conjoined epistemological and ontological dimensions. Among the advantages fitting proffers is visual or 'material anonymity' which Harvey Sacks calls 'doing being ordinary'.[20] Disability theorists are best positioned to reveal the reality of the vulnerability/ power interrelation that shatters the norms of personhood, because they are all too aware of the mythic character of mainstream theories which posit the fully autonomous and independent subject as a necessary precondition for a fully human life, and of success, power, or authority. And yet this is 'real', though it may not be 'true' to take Zillah Eisenstein's phrasing in reverse. For example, the crux of the fractious sex/gender debate in feminism has to do with biological potentiality versus biological determinism.[21] Eisenstein illuminates the terrain of this culturally loaded issue in writing: 'Sex "difference" is someplace between the real and the ideal because the body exists but always through its signs ... the language of sex "difference" may not be all true, but it is real'.[22] But importantly, for those outside the norm, it is in this cognitive identity dissonance between what Garland-Thomson calls 'felt' versus 'attributed identity' that politicization takes root.[23]

Garland-Thomson's misfits concept is material in the sense of a concern with the lived body and also materialist in recognizing the socio-economic (and other) structures that must be navigated in our daily lives, but which we also have a role in sustaining, or making anew. The concept of misfit nicely builds

---

18   Charlotte Witt, *The Metaphysics of Gender.* New York: Oxford University Press, 2011, 131.

19   Garland-Thomson, 'Misfits', 597.

20   Cited in Garland-Thomson, 'Misfits', 596.

21   Zillah Eisenstein, *The Female Body and the Law*, Berkeley: University of California Press, 1988, 96.

22   Eisenstein, *The Female Body and the Law*, 87.

23   Garland-Thomson, 'Misfits', 601.

on O'Brien's biosocial reproduction and the new material feminisms because it emphasizes interactive material/social dynamics rather than positing biological or social determinism, or in Lykke's terms, is a postconstructionist corpo-materialist feminist theory. It remains focused on the interface of (performing) agents and (material) structures in moments of misfitting and fitting without reifying either.[24] 'The dynamism between body and world that produces fits or misfits comes at the spatial and temporal points of encounter between dynamic but *relatively* stable bodies and environments'. Moreover, misfits demonstrate social attitudes as barriers but also material structures, and the concrete effects of this phenomena, namely the privatization (or exclusion from the public sphere) experienced by those who misfit in an ongoing daily way.[25]

Furthermore, misfitting is a universal experience: an ever-present and, in fact, unavoidable situation that affords a unique and beneficial onto-epistemic standpoint.[26] Rather, the 'epistemic status' (not unlike the 'epistemic advantage' of feminist standpoint theory) that misfits confer is necessary and practical for everyone as a way of being and engaging the world and others in it who all, at one point or another, will misfit with the world and experience disability as a result. This radically extends the scope and status of traditional, gendered understandings of the embodiment of vulnerability, and the feminization of care. Furthermore, misfitting brings with it distinct advantages – just as reproduction holds enormous epistemological (and other) richness in patriarchal cultures – that can inform politics and culture (even on a global level) as disability theorists and feminist care ethicists show.[27] Garland-Thomson names 'adaptability, resourcefulness, and subjugated knowledge' as potential advantages of misfitting.[28] For example, sophisticated language cultures have developed from the experience of hearing 'disabilities', and among Garland-Thomson's examples are Claude Monet's development of a more impressionistic style as he became blind, and Jürgen Habermas's revelation that having multiple surgeries positively influenced his intellectual development.

Less dramatically but no less radical, if we take the misfit concept to heart we are always intra-acting with the environment on a micro-level hence such theorization leads to the complex ontology associated with the new material feminisms. Garland-Thomson writes, '*Misfit* ... reflects the shift in feminist theory from an emphasis on the discursive toward the material by centering its analytical focus on the co-constituting relationship between flesh and environment'. The profound and transformative insight related to this theoretical proposition has to do with embodiment that does not amount to another 'wounded attachment' but is a real negotiation of the terms of dualism (including corporeal vulnerability and power)

---

24 Garland-Thomson, 'Misfits', 594.
25 Garland-Thomson, 'Misfits', 594. Emphasis added.
26 Garland-Thomson, 'Misfits', 603.
27 Garland-Thomson, 'Misfits', 604.
28 Garland-Thomson, 'Misfits', 592.

in a sensuous material sense. In this view, existence is a function of a constant process of interaction and change. Agency is fundamentally reconceptualized as in Barad's notion of intra-action rather than inter-action which further departs from the view that we are placed in the world rather than constantly becoming a part of it, and in co-creation with it.[29]

Perhaps most importantly, fitting comes at a distinct cost that is 'complacency about social justice and a desensitizing to material experience;' something that is reflected in a patriarchal society that values control over the body (in its material processes, including reproduction) based on Cartesian mind over body dualism.[30] At the same time I am in agreement with disability theorist Susan Wendell (1988) who reminds us that bodies are not only sources of pleasure to be simply 'reclaimed' for women, and debunks the myth of western medicine that we *can* 'control' our bodies. This is precisely why attendance to differential embodiment, especially those reproductive bodies associated with pure nature, body (instead of mind) and vulnerability (instead of power) is needed especially at a time when it is technologically possible to mediate such differences. Furthermore, embodied reproduction is a uniquely female experience of transmogrification of the (individual) body; an experienced corporeal duality with profound psychological, sociopolitical and philosophical ramifications if seriously engaged. By recognizing the value in the fluctuation of bodily states (our own and others, and over the life course), we also access the powers inseparable from vulnerabilities that women's embodied reproduction symbolizes in patriarchal cultures, seeing in them the kind of intimate yet world-transforming insights they are. Attending to an embodied material engagement with the world, (on a personal as well as a political level), provides the opportunity for negotiating the felt dissonance of our dis/integrated selves in body-phobic cultures which may affect us differently, but fundamentally affect us all.

While the point of difference between feminist postconstructionist epistemologies and postmodern anti-epistemologies is that matter has agency, do new materialist concepts take into account gender and gendered subjectivity? Burfoot provides an incisive analysis of what happens to identity politics 'in the face of biotechnology', in particular, taking issue with some otherwise useful new materialist ideas, because of their abstraction from the specific, sex/gender differentiated experiences of technoscientific tools and practices in patriarchal society. Like I have argued of postmodern theorizations of the body that leave out gender, she writes: 'Barad (and Butler) run the risk of perpetuating a lengthy history of denigration of the body and denial of its continued political experience as gendered. Men do not experience reproductive technologies as women do.

---

29   Karen Barad, 'Posthumanist Performativity: Toward an Understanding of How Matter Comes to Matter', *Signs: Journal of Women in Culture and Society* 28:3 (Spring 2003): 827, 829.

30   Garland-Thomson, 'Misfits', 597.

Period'.[31] She is right. Bodies are birthed, and birth giving bodies are those of women, complex biocultural agents though they may be. Moreover, women's political and economic disabilities are always traceable to what states and societies make of their biological bodies. In describing a body as a site of various inscriptions or emphasizing materiality as emerging from micro-processes, it is easy to lose sight of bodies' own activities and processes, their ontology and agency, pleasures and pains. It is not yet clear how the conceptual advancements of intra-action and the material-discursive will be taken into the practice of science and technology which bear the marks of patriarchal history and ongoing birth appropriation. Furthermore, feminist postconstructionism as a broad 'thinking technology' has not yet been applied to reproductive technologies. On the other hand, the biosocial concept as linked to O'Brien and feminist standpoint has addressed the thorny political and ethical issues surrounding new reproductive technologies. For example, in contemporary feminist theory I have explored the paradox of reproduction in the oppositional responses to NRTs, potentially negotiated in the biosocial equivocal feminist response,[32] as well as in the biosocial dimensions of new material feminisms.

Similarly, new feminist materialisms will have policy implications, even though these have not yet been formulated. Postconstructionist theories comprise a fundamentally biosocial interpretive framework emerging from across a broad range of disciplines (from quantum physics and biology, to sociology) that can be applied to reproductive and other biotechnology policy, but not limited to that. For instance, in Chapter 3 I looked at the Canadian *Assisted Human Reproduction Act (AHRA)* as representing an attempt at the policy level to, at least formally, address the biological and social character of health (in this case reproduction). Such analysis easily extends into competing explanatory variables for illness that build on the understanding of the complex relationship between epistemology and ontology, and mind and body, in the domain of health generally. As part of this, the social determinants of health approach includes discussions of, for example, social and economic disparity as a matter of public health pertinent to the community rather than simply the domain of the isolated individual and is exemplified in feminist responses to new reproductive technologies in Part II, especially the resistance position.

Examining the regulation and implementation of NRTs in Canada, and in comparative perspective, enables an exploration of whether and how health policy takes account of the complex interactions of variables contributing to health that span the biological and social realms, and if not, how it could. For example, such research could examine if and how countries are regulating the use and development of new reproductive and genetic technologies, and how such policies might serve as a guide for other health policy that incorporates the social

---

31   Annette Burfoot, 'Human Remains: Identity Politics in the Face of Biotechnology', *Cultural Critique* 53 (2003): 69.

32   Wendy Brown, 'Wounded Attachments', *Political Theory* 21:3 (1993).

determinants of health. It also enables an assessment of whether and how the use of new reproductive and genetic technology, as currently regulated, reinforce conditions of inequality at both the local and global levels.

Especially interesting in terms of biosocial theory is how changing material (including technological) practices, and social (including legal) practice are related; for example, how has the development of new reproductive and genetic technology both constituted, and been constituted by parallel shifts in thought, and social phenomena? For example, what is the relationship between social and legal understandings of homosexuality, (in gay marriage for instance) and reproductive technology? Furthermore, the global dimension of the biosocial emerges in attending to such phenomena as the retraction of new technologies once introduced, as related to (new) social relations based on entitlement. For example, an international black market in reproductive techniques such as non-medical sex-selection and paid surrogacy arrangements (both of which are prohibited under the AHRA) has been amply documented. Furthermore, international 'medical tourism' raises questions about the way in which the administration and management of health services in one country can have global effects.

In addition, the biosocial concept is evident in critical assessments of the 'geneticization' approach to health at the core of Western culture, which would explore more balanced and biosocial approaches to health care including social, political and environmental policy. Other significant consequences may be a renewed civic participation in health debates and the policy creation process, and greater collaboration amongst fields of study traditionally understood as functioning best autonomously. The transdisciplinarity of the new material feminisms (examined in Part III) provides a working model for alliances among researchers and professionals spanning the social and natural sciences, which has specific importance within the field of healthcare. The problem of translating good theory into good practice is perennial, but feminist postconstructionism is particularly well positioned as a postdiscipline to foster meaningful understandings between researchers, policy makers and health practitioners about the biosocial character of technoscience and health with the goal of better, more effective, policy that brings together the social, environmental, and technological dimensions of reproduction, and health more generally.

Furthermore, and more abstractly – controversial discoveries in medical science like foetomaternal microchimerism can potentially undermine androcentric dualism, and test the limits of the biosocial concept in feminism as well. Aryn Martin explains foetomaternal microchimerism (the continuing, long term genetic interconnection between mothers and children after conception) or 'foetal cell trafficking' as a provocative phenomenon for feminist consideration – especially in light of biology's fraught relationship to feminist theory.[33] Drawing on Barad's similar complication of dichotomous understandings (including nature and

---

33   Aryn Martin, 'Your Mother's Always with You: Material Feminism and Fetomaternal Microchimerism', *Resources for Feminist Research* 33:3–4 (2010): 1.

culture) she explores this phenomenon in terms of 'the entanglement of discourse and materiality' situating it in pro and anti-natal discourse, and as an extension of the messy ways that women fit the individualism of liberal theory at even the biological level.[34] As in O'Brien's work, the notion of biology is significantly complicated as a process rather than conforming to one or the other side of the body/mind dualism, and especially in boldly centralizing the fraught notion of biology, in a sophisticated transdualistic framework.

In a genetics-centric legal framework in which genetic 'mothers' are often privileged over gestational 'surrogates' (explored in Chapter 1), the phenomena of foetomaternal microchimerism may have significant consequences. For example, starting from the perspective of women's material processes of reproduction complicates a simple genetics versus social parenthood model when it comes to legislating surrogacy, even as it may reopen old fault lines of debate between pro- and anti-natalists. For example, it may go without saying that biological motherhood is a fundamentally more complicated proposition than is often reflected in legal judgments but this is especially so when a gestational mother's contribution can be likened to a baby sitter who cares for the child while the genetic mother is unable as was the case in *Johnson v. Calvert* (1991). Microchimerism could provide a challenge that is not just rhetorical, but material as well – which points to nature to contest simple and unitary classification.[35] It is hard to imagine a more profound challenge to feminism's somatophobic Cartesian inheritance than such 'biological being-in-each-other'.[36] At best foetomaternal microchimerism draws attention to the tidy, but false, distinctions amongst physiological/biological, social and genetic aspects of parenthood inaugurated by gestation surrogacy in the mid-1980s. As Goslinga-Roy aptly puts it, such separations are ontologically unstable – especially 'because "genetic" and "biological" aspects of reproduction are also social categories, and all social categories are ultimately embodied processes, deeply implicated in power and history'.[37]

An integral part of this longstanding, disembodiment in theory and practice, is an over-simple and erroneous notion of biology that, in spite of many attempts at re-theorization, has until recently remained stubbornly opposite to politics (or society) in a gendered dualistic framework. In this book I have argued that because 'nature' or 'biology' is a tough test for feminist theory, it has been relegated to the sidelines by many theorists who, especially after the postmodern turn in academia, have been drawn into more ideological or cultural explanations of ongoing androcentrism that leave out the difficult issues of materiality.

---

34 Martin, 'Your Mother's Always with You', 2.

35 Martin, 'Your Mother's Always with You', 7.

36 Martin, 'Your Mother's Always with You', 7.

37 Gillian M. Goslinga-Roy, 'Body Boundaries, Fiction of the Female Self: An Ethnographic Perspective on Power, Feminism, and the Reproductive Technologies', *Feminist Studies* 26:1 (Spring 2000): 113–40, p. 113.

Reactive concepts like biology, are actually politically neutral (if understandably not in feminist studies) but in any case unavoidable and necessary tools for changing the world, as Howie also reflects.[38] What I hope to have shown is that properly understood, materialism again provides the best guide because structural oppression still exists, and we are inescapably embodied and furthermore, have much to gain from embracing the paradoxes of our material engagement with the world, especially for women as potential birth-givers in an age of new reproductive technologies. As such this book is a reflection on feminist science and technology studies as concerned with the notion of communities as knowers and science, in particular, as that hegemonic, yet paradigm shifting community with which we each unavoidably engage as embodied individuals.

In this way we can frame androcentric dualism as a complicated form of epistemic imbalance, or 'epistemic injustice' that indicates the complex, political nature of the interrelationship between knowers. While 'strategic ignorance' or not knowing the marginal perspective is undoubtedly a position of privilege, it is also an epistemic disadvantage as Rosemarie Garland-Thomson shows. For one thing, it leads to a satisfaction with the world hence makes social change less likely. Feminist epistemologists like Nancy Tuana draw attention to the intertwined character of the political and ethical, in highlighting 'the political forces that help direct the research and production of knowledge, shaping patterns of knowledge and ignorance'.[39] While it may seem unrealistic and impractical to ask that people are responsible for what they 'learn how to see' hence know, it is what many feminist social epistemologists have long been arguing for in seeking to '*generate sound and ethical patterns of knowledge and ignorance*' and specifically calling for more democratic processes in shaping these.[40]

As Garland-Thomson plainly puts it, '[a]n embodied engagement with the world is in fact life itself'.[41] Our subjective engagements with the world are bodily mediated which entails crucial differences with one another with very real social, political and ethical implications that should not be reduced to such polar classifications as men versus women, rich versus poor (subject versus object, variously construed) as postmodern and intersectional analysis has shown; but we can pick out patterns of oppression common across dualistic pairings and amongst clustered identity categories that are missed in more discursive formulations of political engagement, and counter hegemony. The ongoing power of feminist standpoint epistemology is in countering hegemonic dualism in patriarchal capitalist cultures. Currently our techno culture, one significant feature of which is new reproductive technologies, is built upon a gender differentiated dualistic foundation that separates mind from body, and form and matter; an androcentric

---

38   Gillian Howie, *Between Feminism and Materialism: A Question of Method*, New York: Palgrave Macmillan 2010, 9.
39   'Feminist Social Epistemology', *Stanford Encyclopedia of Philosophy*, 25.
40   Haraway, 'Situated Knowledges'; 'Feminist Social Epistemology', 25–6.
41   Garland-Thompson, 'Misfits', 600.

approach with patriarchal outcomes, even if not without its paradoxes. In terms of feminist strategizing, however, it is especially important now that the material bases of sex/gender differences (which are a not simply a source of bodily vulnerability, and have been the source of collective feminist organizing) are eroded by NRTs, to recognize commonalities among women while also drawing on theoretical, methodological, and epistemological pluralism that the new material feminisms exemplify.

Bibliography

'Cybernetics', *The New Lexicon Webster's Encyclopedic Dictionary of the English Language*, Canadian Edition, New York: Lexicon Publishers, 1988, 238.

'Calif. Judge Speaks On Issue of Surrogacy', *National Law Journal* 5 (November 1990): 36.

'Dancing Baby', *Macleans*, 12 July 2004, 12.

'Feminist Social Epistemology', *Stanford Encyclopedia of Philosophy*, Stanford University, 2006. Web: http://plato.stanford.edu/entries/feminist-social-epistemology/

Agigian, Amy, *Baby Steps*, Middletown, CT: Wesleyan University Press, 2004.

Ahmed, Sara, 'Open Forum Imaginary Prohibitions: Some Preliminary Remarks on the Founding Gestures of the "New Materialism"', *European Journal of Women's Studies* 15:1 (2008): 23–39.

———, *Strange Encounters: Embodied Others in Post-Coloniality*, New York: Routledge, 2000.

Alaimo, Stacy, and Susan Hekman, eds, *Material Feminisms*, Bloomington: Indiana University Press, 2008.

Alcoff, Linda, 'Cultural Feminism versus Post-Structuralism: The Identity Crisis in Feminist Theory', *Signs: Journal of Women in Culture and Society* 13:3 (1988): 405–36.

———, 'Who's Afraid of Identity Politics?' in *Reclaiming Identity: Realist Theory and the Predicament of Postmodernism*, ed. Paula M.L. Moya and Michael R. Hames-Garcia, California: University of California Press, 2000, 312–44.

Arditti, Rita, 'Commercializing Motherhood', in *The Politics of Motherhood: Activist Voices from Left to Right*, ed. Alexis Jetter, Annelise Orleck and Diana Taylor, Hanover, NH: University Press of New England, 1997, 322–33.

Arditti, Rita, Renate Duelli Klein, and Shelley Minden, eds, *Test-Tube Women: What Future for Motherhood?* London: Pandora Press, 1989.

Aristophanes, Lysistrata, *Aristophanes Four Comedies*, trans. Dudley Fitts, New York: Harcourt, Brace & World, Inc., 1957.

Aristotle, *The Politics of Aristotle*, ed. and trans. Ernest Barker, New York: Oxford University Press, 1958.

Arneil, Barbara, *Politics & Feminism*, Oxford: Blackwell Publishers, 1999.

———, *Politics and Feminism*, USA: Wiley, 1999, 188.

Arney, William R., *Power and the Profession of Obstetrics*, Chicago: University of Chicago Press, 1982.

Asberg, Cecilia, 'Enter Cyborg: Tracing the Historiography and Ontological Turn of Feminist Technoscience Studies', *International Journal of Feminist Technoscience* 1:1 (2010).

Asberg, Cecilia and Nina Lykke, 'Feminist Technoscience Studies', *European Journal of Women's Studies* 17:4 (2010): 299–305.

Atwood, Margaret, *The Handmaid's Tale*, Toronto: Seal Books, 1986.

Augustine, *Confessions*, trans. R.S. Pine-Coffin, Middlesex, England: Penguin Books Ltd, 1975.

Bailey, M.E, 'Foucauldian Feminism: Contesting Bodies, Sexuality and Identity', in *Up Against Foucault: Explorations of Some Tensions between Foucault and Feminism*, ed. Caroline Ramazanoglu, London: Routledge, 1993, 99–122.

Baillairge, Melanie, 'Paula Pan Syndrome: A Thirtysomething wonders if you have to be a mom to really feel like a woman', *Elle Canada* (May 2002): 73–4.

Baird, Patricia, 'New Reproductive Technologies: The Canadian Perspective', *Women's Health Issues* 6:3 (1996): 156–65.

Barad, Karen, 'Getting Real: Technoscientific Practices and the Materialization of Reality', *Differences: A Journal of Feminist Cultural Studies* 10:2 (1998): 87–128.

———, 'Meeting the Universe Halfway: Realism and Social Constructivism without Contradiction', in *Feminism, Science and the Philosophy of Science*, ed. Lynn Hankinson Nelson and Jack Nelson, Dordrecht, the Netherlands: Kluwer, 1997.

———, *Meeting the Universe Halfway: Quantum Physics and the Entanglement of Matter and Meaning*, Durham and London: Duke University Press, 2007.

———, 'Posthumanist Performativity: Toward an Understanding of How Matter Comes to Matter', *Signs: Journal of Women in Culture and Society* 28:3 (2003), 801–31.

Barr, Marleen S., *Lost In Space: Probing Feminist Science Fiction and Beyond*, Chapel Hill: University of North Carolina Press, 1993.

Barthes, Roland, *Image, Music, Text*, ed. and trans. Stephen Heath, New York: Hill and Wang, 1977.

Bartkowski, Frances, 'Epistemic Drift in Foucault', in *Feminism and Foucault Reflections on Resistance*, ed. Irene Diamond and Lee Quinby, Boston: Northeastern University Press, 1988, 43–58.

Basen, Gwynne, Margrit Eichler and Abby Lippman, eds, *Misconceptions: The Social Construction of Choice and the New Reproductive and Genetic Technologies*, Vol. 1, Prescott, Ontario: Voyageur Publishing, 1993.

———, *Misconceptions: The Social Construction of Choice and the New Reproductive and Genetic Technologies*, Vol. 2, Prescott, Ontario: Voyageur Publishing, 1994.

Beasley, Chris, and Carol Bacchi, 'Citizen Bodies: Embodying Citizens – a Feminist Analysis', *International Feminist Journal of Politics* 2:3 (2000): 337–58.

Bennett, Rebecca, 'Is Reproduction Women's Business? How Should We Regulate Regarding Stored Embryos, Posthumous Pregnancy, Ectogenesis and Male Pregnancy?', *Studies in Ethics, Law, and Technology* 2:3 (2008).

Berer, Marge, 'Breeding Conspiracies: Feminism and the New Reproductive Technologies', *Trouble and Strife* 9 (1986): 29–35.

Bessner, Ronda, 'State Intervention in Pregnancy', *Misconceptions*, Vol. 2, ed. Gwynne Basen, Margrit Eichler and Abby Lippman, Ontario: Voyageur Publishing, 1994, 171–80.

Bimber, Bruce, 'Measuring the Gender Gap on the Internet', *Social Science Quarterly* 81: 3 (2000): 868–76.

Birke, Lynda, *Feminism and the Biological Body*, Edinburgh: Edinburgh University Press, 1999.

———, *Women, Feminism and Biology: The Feminist Challenge*, Brighton, UK: Wheatsheaf Books, 1986.

Birke, Lynda and Cecilia Asberg, 'Biology is a Feminist Issue: Interview with Lynda Birke', *European Journal of Women's Studies* 17:4 (2010): 413–23.

Blaze, Alex, 'New Jersey Court Decides Against Gestational Surrogacy Contracts', *The Bilerico Project*, 5 January 2010.

Bordo, Susan, 'Feminism, Foucault and the Politics of the Body', in *Up Against Foucault*, ed. Caroline Ramazanoglu, London: Routledge, 1993, 179–202.

———, 'Feminism, Postmodernism, and Gender-Scepticism', in *Feminism/Postmodernism*, ed. Linda J. Nicholson, New York: Routledge, 1990, 133–57.

Boucher, Joanne, 'Male Power and Contract Theory: Hobbes and Locke in Carole Pateman's The Sexual Contract', *Canadian Journal of Political Science* 36:1 (2003): 23–38.

Braidotti, Rosi, 'Cyberfeminism with a Difference', *Utrecht University*, 16 September 2003: http://www.let.uu.nl/womens_studies/rosi/cyberfem.htm

———, *Patterns of Dissonance: A Study of Women in Contemporary Philosophy*, Cambridge: Polity Press, 1991.

———, '"Teratologies"', in *Deleuze and Feminist Theory*, ed. Ian Buchanan Claire Colebrook, Edinburgh: Edinburgh University Press, 2000, 56–72.

Brayton, Jennifer, *Cyberfeminism as New Theory*, http://www.unb.ca/web/PAR-L/win/cyberfem.htm. Accessed 17 September 2003.

Brodie, Janine, *Politics on the Margins: Restructuring and the Canadian Women's Movement*, Halifax, Canada: Fernwood Publishing, 1995.

Brodribb, Somer, *Nothing Mat(t)ers: A Feminist Critique of Postmodernism*, Toronto: James Lorimer and Company, 1993.

———, 'Off the Pedestal and onto the Block? Motherhood, Reproductive Technologies, and the Canadian State', *Canadian Journal of Women and the Law* 1:2 (1986): 407–23.

Brown, Wendy, 'Wounded Attachments', *Political Theory* 21:3 (1993): 390–410.

Burchell, Graham, Colin Gordon and Peter Miller, eds, *The Foucault Effect: Studies in Governmentality*, Chicago: University of Chicago Press, 1991.

Burfoot, Annette, 'Feminist Technoscience: A Solution to Theoretic Conundrums and the Wane of Feminist Politics?' *Resources for Feminist Research* 33:3 (2010): 71–85.

———, 'Human Remains: Identity Politics in the Face of Biotechnology', *Cultural Critique* 53 (2003): 47–71.

———, 'In-Appropriation – A Critique of "Proceed with Care: Final Report of the Royal Commission on New Reproductive Technologies"', *Women's Studies International Forum* 18:4 (1995): 499–506.

———, 'Revisiting Mary O'Brien – Reproductive Consciousness and Liquid Maternity', Marxisms and Feminisms on the Edge, Society for Socialist Studies: Annual Meeting. Victoria, BC, 5–7 June 2013. Paper Presentation.

Butler, Judith, *Bodies That Matter: On the Discursive Limits of 'Sex'*, New York: Routledge, 1993.

———, 'Contingent Foundations', in *Twentieth Century Political Theory: A Reader*, ed. Stephen Eric Bronner, New York: Routledge, 1997, 248–58.

———, 'Gender as Performance', in *A Critical Sense: Interviews with Intellectuals*, ed. P. Osborne. London; New York: Routledge, 1996.

———, *Gender Trouble: Feminism and the Subversion of Identity*, New York: Routledge, 1990.

———, *The Psychic Life of Power: Theories in Subjection*, Stanford, California: California University Press, 1997.

Cairns, Huntington, and Edith Hamilton, eds, *The Collected Dialogues of Plato*, Bollingen Series LXXI, Princeton, NJ: Princeton University Press, 1989.

The Canadian Law Reform Commission, *Crimes Against the Fetus: Working Paper 58*, Department of Justice, Canada, 1989.

Carr, Nicholas, *The Shallows: How the Internet is Changing the Way We Read, Think and Remember*, London: Atlantic Books, 2010.

Chanter, Tina, 'Postmodern Subjectivity', in *A Companion to Feminist Philosophy*, ed. Alison Jaggar and Iris Marion Young, Malden, MA: Blackwell, 1998, 263–72.

Cheal, David, 'Authority and Incredulity: Sociology between Modernism and Postmodernism', *Canadian Journal of Sociology* 15:3 (1989): 129–47.

Chodorow, Nancy, *The Reproduction of Mothering*, London: University of California Press, 1978.

Clarke, Adele, *Disciplining Reproduction: Modernity, American Life Sciences, and the 'Problems of Sex'*, California: University of California Press, 1998.

Clynes, Manfred E., and Nathan S. Kline, 'Cyborgs in Space', in *The Cyborg Handbook*, ed. Chris Hables Gray, Heidi J. Figueroa-Sarriera, and Steven Montor, New York and London: Routledge, 1995, 29–34.

Colebatch, H.K., 'Government and Governmentality: Using Multiple Approaches to the Analysis of Government', *Australian Journal of Political Science* 37:3 (2002): 417–35.

Colebrook, Claire, 'On Not Becoming Man: The Materialist Politics of Unactualized Potential', in *Material Feminism*, ed. Susan Hekman, Stacy Alaimo, Bloomington: Indiana University Press, 2008, 73–5.

Colker, Ruth, *Abortion & Dialogue*, Bloomington: Indiana University Press, 1992.

———, 'An Equal Protection Analysis of United States Reproductive Health Policy: Gender, Race, Age, and Class', *Duke Law Journal* (1991): 324–64.

———, 'The Practice of Theory', *Northwestern University Law Review* 87 (1993): 1273–85.

———, *Pregnant Men: Practice, Theory, and the Law*, Bloomington: Indiana University Press, 1994.

Collins, Francoise, 'Philosophical Differences', in *A History of Women: Toward a Cultural Identity in the Twentieth Century*, ed. Francois Thebaud, Cambridge, MA: Harvard University Press, 1994, 261–96.

Connell, R.W., 'The State, Gender and Sexual Politics: Theory and Appraisal', in *Power/Gender: Social Relations in Theory and Practice*, ed. H. Lorraine Radtke and Henderikus J. Stam, London and Thousand Oaks, CA: Sage Publications, 1994, 507–44.

Coole, Diana, *Women in Political Theory: From Ancient Misogyny to Contemporary Feminism*, New York: Harvester Wheatsheaf, 1993.

Coole, Diana and Samantha Frost, eds, *New Materialisms: Ontology, Agency, and Politics*, Durham and London: Duke University Press, 2010.

Corea, Gena, *The Mother Machine: Reproductive Technologies from Artificial Insemination to Artificial Wombs*, New York: Harper and Row, 1985.

Costa, Gabrielle, 'Backdown On "Psychological Infertility"', *The Age*, 21 November 2001.

Dallery, Arleen B, 'Sexual Embodiment: Beauvoir and French Feminism (*ecriture feminine*)', *Women's Studies International Forum* 8:3 (1985): 197–202.

Danaher, Geoff, Tony Schirato, and Jen Webb, *Understanding Foucault*, Australia: Allen and Unwin, 2000.

Daniels, Cynthia, 'Between Fathers and Fetuses: The Social Construction of Male Reproduction and the Politics of Fetal Harm', *Signs: Journal of Women in Culture and Society* 22:3 (1997): 579–616.

Daniels, Jessie, 'Rethinking Cyberfeminism(s): Race, Gender, and Embodiment', *WSQ: Women's Studies Quarterly* 37:1–2 (2009): 101–24.

Daston, Lorraine, 'Enlightenment Fears, Fears of Enlightenment', in *What's Left of Enlightenment? A Postmodern Question*, ed. Keither Michael Baker and Peter Hanns Reill, Stanford, CA: Stanford University Press, 2001, 116–28.

Davis, Noela, 'New Materialism and Feminism's Anti-Biologism: A Response to Sara Ahmed', in *European Journal of Women's Studies* 16:1 (2009): 67–80.

Davis-Floyd, Robbie E., 'The Technocratic Body and the Organic Body: Cultural Models for Women's Birth Choices', in *Knowledge and Society: The Anthology of Science and Technology*, Vol. 9, ed. David Hess and Linda Layen, Greenwich, CT: JAI Press Inc., 1992, 59–93.

————, 'The Technocratic, Humanistic, and Holistic Models of Birth', *International Journal of Obstetrics and Gynecology* 75:1 (2001): S5–S23.

De Beauvoir, Simone, *The Second Sex*, trans. H.M. Parshley, New York: Vintage Books, 1989.

Dean, Mitchell, *Governmentality: Power and Rule in Modern Society*, London: Sage, 1999.

Deveaux, Monique, 'Feminism and Empowerment: A Critical Reading of Foucault', in *Feminist Interpretations of Michel Foucault*, ed. Susan J. Hekman, University Park, PA: Pennsylvania State University Press, 1996, 211–38.

Dhruvarajan, Vanaja and Jill Vickers, eds, *Gender, Race, and Nation: A Global Perspective*, Toronto: University of Toronto Press, 2002.

Diamond, Irene, *Fertile Ground: Women, Earth, and the Limits of Control*, Boston: Beacon Press, 1994.

Diamond, Irene, and Lee Quinby, 'Introduction', in *Feminism and Foucault: Reflections on Resistance*, ed. Irene Diamond and Lee Quinby, Boston: Northeastern University Press, 1988, ix–xx.

Dobson (Litigation Guardian of) v. Dobson, 1997, 143 Dominion Law Revue. (4th) 189.

Ehrenreich, Barbara, and Deirdre English, *Witches, Midwives, and Nurses: A History of Women Healers*, Detroit: Black and Red, 1973.

Eisenstein, Zillah R., *The Female Body and the Law*, Berkeley: University of California Press, 1988.

————, *The Radical Future of Liberal Feminism*, Boston: Northeastern University Press, 1981.

Eisler, Riane, *The Chalice and the Blade: Our History, Our Future*, Cambridge, MA: Harper & Row, 1987.

Elshtain, Jean Bethke, *Public Man, Private Woman: Women in Social and Political Thought*, Princeton, NJ: Princeton University Press, 1981.

Epstein, Rachel, *Who's Your Daddy: And Other Writings on Queer Parenting*, 1st edn, Toronto: Sumach Press, 2009.

Fausto-Sterling, Anne, 'The Bare Bones of Sex: Part I, Sex & Gender', *Signs*, 30:2 (2005): 1491–528.

————, *Sexing the Body: Gender Politics and the Construction of Sexuality*, New York: Basic Books, 2000.

Fine, Michelle, and Adrienne Asch, 'Who Owns the Womb?' *The Women's Review of Books* 2:8 (1985): 8–10.

————, eds, *Women with Disabilities: Essays in Psychology, Culture, and Politics*, Philadelphia: Temple University Press, 1988.

Finger, A, 'Claiming all of our Bodies: Reproductive Rights and Disability', in *Test-Tube Women: What Future for Motherhood?*, ed. R. Arditti, R.D. Klein and S. Minden, London: Pandora Press, 1984, 281–97.

————, *Past Due: A Story of Disability, Pregnancy and Birth*, Seattle: Seal Press, 1990.

Firestone, Shulamith, *The Dialectic of Sex: The Case for Feminist Revolution*, New York: Quill William Morrow, 1970.

Forman, Frieda Johles, and Caoran Sowton, eds, *Taking Our Time: Feminist Perspectives on Temporality*, Oxford: Pergamon Press, 1989.

Foucault, Michel, 'The Birth of Biopolitics', in *Ethics: Subjectivity and Truth*, ed. Paul Rabinow, New York: The New Press, 1997, 73–9.

———, 'Body/Power', in *Power/Knowledge: Selected Interviews and Other Writings 1972–1977*, ed. Colin Gordon, trans. Colin Gordon, Leo Marshall, John Mepham and Kate Soper, Brighton: The Harvester Press, 1980, 55–62.

———, 'Clarifications on the Question of Power', in *Foucault Live: Collected Interviews, 1961–1984*, ed. Sylvère Lotringer, New York: Semiotext(e), 1996, 255–63.

———, 'The Eye of Power', in *Foucault Live: Collected Interviews, 1961–1984*, ed. Sylvère Lotringer, New York: Semiotext(e), 1996, 226–40.

———, 'Governmentality', in *The Foucault Effect: Studies in Governmentality*, ed. Graham Burchell, Colin Gordon and Peter Miller, Chicago: University of Chicago Press, 1991, 87–104.

———, *The History of Sexuality Vol. 1: An Introduction*, trans. Robert Hurley, New York: Vintage, 1990.

———, *The History of Sexuality Vol. 2: The Use of Pleasure*, trans. Robert Hurley, New York: Vintage Books, 1990.

———, *The History of Sexuality Vol. 3: The Care of the Self*, trans. Robert Hurley, New York: Vintage Books, 1990.

———, 'Power Affects the Body', in *Foucault Live: Collected Interviews, 1961–1984*, ed. Sylvère Lotringer, New York: Semiotext(e), 1996, 207–13.

———, 'Sex, Power and the Politics of Identity', in *Foucault Live: Collected Interviews, 1961–1984*, ed. Sylvère Lotringer, New York: Semiotext(e), 1996, 382–90.

———, 'Society Must Be Defended', in *Ethics: Subjectivity and Truth*, ed. Paul Rabinow, New York: The New Press, 1997, 59–66.

———, 'Two Lectures', in *Power/Knowledge: Selected Interviews and Other Writings 1972–1977*, ed. Colin Gordon, trans. Colin Gordon, Leo Marshall, John Mepham and Kate Soper, Brighton: The Harvester Press, 1980, 78–108.

Franklin, Sarah, *Embodied Progress: A Cultural Account of Assisted Conception*, London: Routledge, 1997.

———, 'Life Itself: Global Nature and the Genetic Imaginary' in *Global Nature, Global Culture*, ed. Sarah Franklin, Celia Lury and Jackie Stacey, Trowbridge, Wiltshire, UK: The Cromwell Press, 2000, 188–227.

———, 'Postmodern Procreation: A Cultural Account of Assisted Reproduction', in *Conceiving the New World Order: The Global Politics of Reproduction*, ed. Faye D. Ginsburg and Rayna Rapp, Berkeley: University of California Press, 1995, 323–45.

Fuss, Diana, *Essentially Speaking: Feminism, Nature and Difference*, New York: Routledge, 1989.

Galst, Liz, and Joan Hilty, 'Lesbians with Strollers: The Gaybie Boom on Wheels', *Ms.* XIII (Spring 2003): 17–18.

Gamble, Sarah, ed., *The Routledge Critical Dictionary of Feminism and Postfeminism*, New York: Routledge, 2000.

Garland-Thomson, Rosemarie, 'Misfits: A Feminist Materialist Disability Concept', *Hypatia* 26:3 (Summer, 2011): 591–601.

Gearey, Jennifer, 'Putting a Face to the Unborn: The Latest Ultrasound Technology Comes Alive in Ottawa', *Ottawa Citizen*, 5 June 2004, A14.

Gevenson, Tavi, 'Still Figuring it Out' TedxTeen Talk, 31 March 2012: http://tedxteen.com/talks/tedxteen-2012/112-tavi-gevinson-still-figuring-it-out.

Gibson, William, *Neuromancer*, New York: Ace Books, 1984.

Gilligan, Carol, *In a Different Voice*, Cambridge, MA: Harvard University Press, 1982.

Ginsburg, Faye D., and Rayna Rapp, eds, *Conceiving the New World Order: The Global Politics of Reproduction*, California: University of California Press, 1995.

Glossary of Terms, 'Dialectics', *Encyclopedia of Marxism*, Marxist Internet Archive, 1999. Web.

Goslinga-Roy, Gillian M., 'Body Boundaries, Fiction of the Female Self: An Ethnographic Perspective on Power, Feminism, and the Reproductive Technologies', *Feminist Studies* 26:1 (Spring 2000): 113–40, p. 113.

Government Services Canada, *Proceed With Care: Final Report of the Royal Commission on New Reproductive Technologies*, Ottawa, Canada: Minister of Government Services Canada, 1993.

Grant, Judith, *Fundamental Feminism*, London: Routledge, 1994.

Greer, Germaine, *The Whole Woman*, Toronto: Doubleday, 1999.

Grosz, Elizabeth, *Volatile Bodies: Toward a Corporeal Feminism*, Bloomington: Indiana University Press, 1994.

Gustafsson, Siv, 'Having Kids Later: Economic Analyses for Industrialized Countries', *Review of Economics of the Household* 3 (2005): 5–16.

Gutting, Gary, *Foucault: A Very Short Introduction*, New York: Oxford University Press, 2005.

Hadd, Wendi, 'A Womb with A View: Women as Mothers and the Discourse of the Body', *Berkeley Journal of Sociology* 36 (1991): 165–75.

Hammarstrom, Matz 'On the Concepts of Transaction and Intra-action', *The Third Nordic Pragmatism Conference*. Uppsala, 1–2 June 2010, 9–10. Conference paper.

Hansen, Mark, 'Surrogacy Contract Upheld: Calif. Supreme Court says such agreements don't violate public policy', *American Bar Association Journal* (August 1993): 34.

Haraway, Donna, 'A Cyborg Manifesto: Science, Technology, and Socialist-Feminism in the Late Twentieth Century', in *Simians, Cyborgs, and Women: The Reinvention of Nature*, ed. Donna Haraway, New York: Routledge, 1991, 149–81.

————, 'A Cyborg Manifesto: Science, Technology, and Socialist-Feminism in the 1980s' in *The Haraway Reader*, New York: Routledge, 2004.

————, *Feminism and Methodology*, Milton Keynes: Open University Press, 1987.

————, *Simians, Cyborgs, and Women: The Reinvention of Nature*, New York: Routledge, 1991.

————, Situated Knowledges: The Science Question in Feminism and the Privilege of Partial Perspective', *Feminist Studies* 14:3 (1988): 575–99.

————, 'Situated Knowledges: The Science Question in Feminism and the Privilege of Partial Perspective' in *Simians, Cyborgs and Women. The Reinvention of Nature*, ed. Donna Haraway, London: Free Association Books, 1991, 183–201.

————, *Whose Science? Whose Knowledge?* Milton Keynes: Open University Press, 1991.

Harding, Sandra, *The Science Question in Feminism*, Milton Keynes: Open University Press, 1986.

Hartland, Edwin Sidney, *Primitive Paternity: The Myth of Supernatural Birth in Relation to the History of the Family*, vols 1 and 2, New York: B. Blom, 1971.

Hartouni, Valerie, *Cultural Conceptions: On Reproductive Technologies and The Remaking of Life*, Minneapolis: University of Minnesota Press, 1997.

Hartsock, Nancy, 'The Feminist Standpoint: Developing the Ground for a Specifically Feminist Historical Materialism' in *Discovering Reality*, ed. Sandra Harding and Merrill Hintikka, Boston: D. Reidel, 1983, 283–310.

————, *The Feminist Standpoint Revisited & Other Essays*, Boulder, CO: Westview Press, 1998.

————, 'Foucault on Power: A Theory for Women?' in *Feminism/Postmodernism*, ed. Linda J. Nicholson, New York: Routledge, 1990, 157–75.

————, 'Mary O'Brien's Feminist Theory', *Canadian Woman Studies* 18:4 (1999): 61–8.

————, *Money, Sex and Power*, New York: Longman, 1983.

Health Canada, *Assisted Human Reproduction Legislation Receives Approval of Senate:* <www.hcsc.ca/english/media/releases/2004/2004_10.htm> Accessed 20 March 2004.

Hearne, Jeff, 'Mary O'Brien ... Certainly the Most Important Single Intellectual Influence ... ', *Canadian Woman Studies* 18:4 (Winter 1999): 13–17.

Hekman, Susan J., *Feminist Interpretations of Michel Foucault*, University Park, PA: Pennsylvania State University Press, 1996.

————, *Moral Voices Moral Selves: Carol Gilligan and Feminist Moral Theory*, University Park, PA: Pennsylvania State University Press, 1995.

Hemmings, Clare, 'Generational Dilemmas: A Response to Iris van der Tuin's "'Jumping Generations': on Second- and Third-wave Feminist Epistemology'", *Australian Feminist Studies* 24:59 (2009): 33–7.

————, *Why Stories Matter: The Political Grammar of Feminist Theory*, Durham, NC: Duke University Press, 2011.

Heyes, Cressida, 'Identity Politics', *Stanford Encyclopedia of Philosophy*, Stanford University, 2002. Web: http://plato.stanford.edu/entries/identity-politics/

Hird, Myra J., 'Feminist Matters: New Materialist Considerations of Sexual Difference', *Feminist Theory* 5:2 (2004): 223–32.

Hirshman, Linda R., 'Looking to the Future, Feminism Has to Focus', *The Washington Post*, 8 June 2008: http://www.washingtonpost.com/wp-dyn/content/article/2008/06/06/AR2008060603494.html

Hobbes, Thomas, *Body, Man, and Citizen*, New York: The Macmillan Company, 1967.

———, *The Citizen: Philosophical Rudiments Concerning Government and Society*, ed. Bernard Gert, Garden City, NY: Doubleday, 1972.

———, *De Cive*, Introduction and ed. Sterling Lamprecht, New York: Appleton-Century-Crofts, 1949.

———, *Leviathan*, New York: Penguin, 1985.

———, *On the Citizen*, ed. Richard Tuck and Michael Silverthorne, Cambridge: Cambridge University Press, 1998.

Holla-Bhar, Radha, and Vandana Shiva, 'Piracy by Patent: The Case of the Neem Tree', in *The Case Against the Global Economy And For a Turn Toward the Local*, ed. Jerry Mander and Edward Goldsmith, San Francisco: Sierra Club Books, 1996, 146–59.

Hornstein, Francie, 'Children by Donor Insemination: A New Choice for Lesbians', in *Test-Tube Women: What Future for Motherhood*, ed. Rita Arditti, Renate Duelli Klein and Shelley Minden, London: Pandora Press, 1989.

Howie, Gillian, *Between Feminism and Materialism: A Question of Method*, New York: Palgrave Macmillan 2010.

Howson, Alexandra, *Embodying Gender*, London: Sage Publishers, 2005.

Hubbard, Ruth, Mary Sue Henifin and Barbara Fried, eds, *Biological Woman – The Convenient Myth: A Collection of Feminist Essays and a Comprehensive Bibliography*, Cambridge, MA: Schenkman Publishing Co., 1982.

Jackson, Stevi, 'Why a Materialist Feminism is (Still) Possible – and Necessary', *Women's Studies International Forum* 24:3–4 (2001): 283–93.

Jameson, Frederic, *Postmodernism, or The Cultural Logic of Late Capitalism*, New York: Verso, 1993.

Jervis, John, *Exploring the Modern: Patterns of Western Culture and Civilization*, Oxford: Blackwell, 1998.

Jetter, Alexis, Annelise Orleck and Diana Taylor, eds, *The Politics of Motherhood: Activist Voices from Left to Right*, Hanover and London: University Press of New England, 1997.

Jhappan, Radha, 'Post-Modern Race and Gender Essentialism or a Post-Mortem of Scholarship', *Studies in Political Economy* 51 (Fall 1996): 15–64.

Johnson v. Calvert, 1993, 5 California Reports, 4th 84.

Johnson, Candace, 'The Political 'Nature' of Pregnancy and Childbirth', *The Canadian Journal of Political Science*, 41:4 (December 2008): 889–913.

Kallianes, Virginia, and Phyllis Rubenfeld, 'Disabled Women and Reproductive Rights', *Disability & Society* 12:2 (1997): 203–21.

Kaplan, Ann E., and Susan Squier, eds, *Playing Dolly: Technocultural Formations, Fantasies, and Fictions of Assisted Reproduction*, New Brunswick, NJ: Rutgers University Press, 1999.

Kaplan, D., 'Disability Rights Perspectives on Reproductive Technologies and Public Policy', in *Reproductive Laws for the 1990s*, ed. Nadine Taub and Sherrill Cohen, New Brunswick: Rutgers University, 1988, 241–7.

Katz-Rothman, Barbara, 'The Meanings of Choice in Reproductive Technology', in *Test-Tube Women: What Future for Motherhood?*, ed. Rita Arditti, Renate Duelli Klein and Shelley Minden, London: Pandora Press, 1984, 23–34.

Kaw, Eugene, 'Medicalization of Racial Features', in *The Politics of Women's Bodies: Sexuality, Appearance and Behavior*, ed. Rose Weitz, 167–83, New York: Oxford University Press, 1998.

Kempley, Rita, 'Prenatal Pictures: Womb for Trouble? A growing trend has some worried about this use of ultrasound', *The Washington Post*, 18 August 2003, 1.

Kimbrell, Andrew, 'Biocolonization: The Patenting of Life and the Global Market in Body Parts', in *The Case Against the Global Economy And For a Turn Toward the Local*, ed. Jerry Mander and Edward Goldsmith, San Francisco: Sierra Club Books, 1996, 131–45.

King, Warren, and Carol M. Ostrom, 'Clinic Split over Fertility Help for Single Women, Lesbians', *Seattle Times*, 12 November 1993.

Kneen, Brewster, *Farmageddon: Food and the Culture of Biotechnology*, Gabriola Island, BC: New Society Publishers, 1999.

Kneen, Cathleen, 'Biotechnology: A Woman's Business', *Women & Environments International* 44–45 (1998): 28–31.

Kolmar, Wendy and Frances Bartkowski, eds, *Feminist Theory: A Reader*, Mountain View, CA: Mayfield Publishing Company, 2000.

Kruks, Sonia, 'Simone de Beauvoir: Engaging Discrepant Materialisms', in *New Materialisms: Ontology, Agency, and Politics*, ed. Diana Coole and Samantha Frost, Durham and London: Duke University Press, 2010.

Laqueur, Thomas, *Making Sex: Body and Gender from the Greeks to Freud*, Cambridge, MA: Harvard University Press, 1992.

Latour, Bruno, *We Have Never Been Modern*, trans. Catherine Porter, Cambridge, MA: Harvard University Press, 1993.

Lazaro, Reyes, 'Feminism and Motherhood: O'Brien vs. Beauvoir', *Hypatia* 1:2 (Fall 1986): 87–102.

Legge M., R. Fitzgerald and N. Frank, 'A Retrospective Study of New Zealand Case Law Involving Assisted Reproduction Technology and the Social Recognition of 'New' Family', *Human Reproduction* 22:1 (2007): 17–25.

Lerner, Gerda, *The Creation of Patriarchy*, New York: Oxford University Press, 1986.

Lie, Merete, 'Science as Father? Sex and Gender in the Age of Reproductive Technologies', in *The European Journal of Women's Studies* 9:4 (2002): 381–399.

Lippman, Abby, 'C-section fight does a U-turn' *Globe and Mail*, 3 March 2004, A21.

———, 'Worrying – and Worrying About – the Geneticization of Reproduction and Health', in *Misconceptions: The Social Construction of Choice and the New Reproductive and Genetic Technologies*, Vol. 1, ed. Gwynne Basen, Margrit Eichler and Abby Lippman, Prescott, Ontario: Voyageur Publishing, 1993, 39–65.

Lublin, Nancy, *Pandora's Box: Feminism Confronts Reproductive Technology*, Lanham, MD: Rowman and Littlefield Publishers, 1998.

Lykke, Nina, *Feminist Studies: A Guide to Intersectional Theory, Methodology, and Writing*, New York: Routledge, 2010.

———, 'The Timeliness of Post-Constructionism', *NORA – Nordic Journal of Feminist and Gender Research* 18:2 (2010): 131–36.

Lyotard, Jean-Francois, 'Introduction to the Postmodern Condition: A Report on Knowledge', in *Twentieth Century Political Theory: A Reader*, ed. Stephen Eric Bronner, New York: Routledge, 1997, 239–41.

MacKinnon, Catherine, 'Feminism, Marxism, Method and the State: An Agenda for Theory', in *Feminist Theory: A Critique of Ideology*, ed. Nannerl O. Keohane, Michelle Z. Rosaldo and Barbara C. Gelpi, Brighton: Harvester, 1982, 1–30.

———, *Feminism Unmodified*, Boston: Harvard University Press, 1987.

———, 'From Practice to Theory, or what is a White Woman Anyway?' *Yale Journal of Law and Feminism* 4 (1991): 13–22.

———, *Toward a Feminist Theory of the State*, Boston: Harvard University Press, 1989.

———, 'Reflections on Sex Equality under Law', *Yale Law Journal* 100 (1991): 1281–328.

McLuhan, Marshall, *Understanding Media: The Extensions of Man*, London: Routledge, 1967.

McNeil, Maureen. Keynote presentation opening of the Posthumanities Hub. Linkoping University, 6 October 2009.

McTeer, Maureen, *In My Own Name: A Memoir*, Canada: Random House, 2003.

McVeigh, Karen, 'Study finds widespread 'criminalisation of pregnancy' in US institutions', *The Guardian*, 15 January 2013: http://www.theguardian.com/world/2013/jan/15/criminalisation-pregnancy-women-study

Mahowald, Mary Briody, ed., *Philosophy of Woman: An Anthology of Classic to Current Concepts*, 3rd edn, Indianapolis, IN: Hackett Publishing Company, Inc., 1994.

Makus, Ingrid, *Women, Politics and Reproduction: The Liberal Legacy*, Toronto: University of Toronto Press, 1996.

Mander, Jerry, 'Technologies of Globalization', *The Case Against the Global Economy And For a Turn Toward the Local*, ed. Jerry Mander and Edward Goldsmith, San Francisco: Sierra Club Books, 1996, 344–59.

Markens, Susan, *Surrogate Motherhood and the Politics of Reproduction*, Berkeley: University of California Press, 2007.

Martin, Aryn, 'Your Mother's Always with You: Material Feminism and Fetomaternal Microchimerism', *Resources for Feminist Research* 33:3–4 (2010), 31–6.

Martin, Jane Roland, 'Methodological Essentialism, False Difference, and Other Dangerous Traps', *Signs* 19:3 (1994): 630–57.

Martin, Linda and Gillian Howie, 'Breaking Feminist Waves' Series Foreword in *Between Feminism and Materialism: A Question of Method*, ed. Gillian Howie, New York: Palgrave Macmillan 2010.

Marx, Anthony W., *Making Race and Nation: A Comparison of South Africa, the United States, and Brazil*, New York: Cambridge University Press, 1998.

Marx, Karl and Friedrich Engels, 'Preface to the Critique of Political Economy', Selected Works, London: Lawrence and Wishart, 1968.

Marzani, Carl, *The Open Marxism of Antonio Gramsci*, trans. C. Marzani, New York: Cameron Associates.

Matthews, Gwyneth F., *Voices from the Shadows: Women with Disabilities Speak Out*, Toronto: The Women's Press, 1983.

Menzies, Heather, 'Technological Time and Infertility', *Canadian Woman Studies* 18:4 (1999): 69–74.

———, *Canada in the Global Village*, Ottawa: Carleton University Press, 1997.

———, *No Time: Stress and the Crisis of Modern Life*, Vancouver, Canada: Douglas & McIntyre Ltd, 2005.

Merchant, Carolyn, 'Ecofeminism and Feminist Theory', in *Environmental Ethics*, ed. Michael Boylan, Upper Saddle River, NJ: Prentice Hall, 2001, 76–83.

———, 'Mining the Earth's Womb', in *Philosophy of Technology: The Technological Condition: An Anthology*, ed. Robert C. Scharff and Val Dusek, Malden, MA: Blackwell Publishers, 2003, 417–28.

———, *The Death of Nature: Women, Ecology and the Scientific Revolution*, San Francisco: Harper San Francisco, 1980.

Merck, Mandy and Stella Sandford, *Further Adventures of the Dialectic of Sex: Critical Essays on Shulamith Firestone*, Basingstoke: Palgrave Macmillan, 2010.

Messing, Karen, and Gail Ouellette, 'A Prevention Oriented Approach to Reproductive Problems: Identifying Environmental Effects', in *Misconceptions: The Social Construction of Choice and the New Reproductive and Genetic Technologies*, Vol. 1, ed. Gwynne Basen, Margrit Eichler and Abby Lippman, Prescott, Ontario: Voyageur Publishing, 1993.

Mies, Maria, 'Liberating Women, Liberating Knowledge: Reflections on Two Decades of Feminist Action Research', *Atlantis* 21:1 (1996): 10–24.

————, 'New Reproductive Technologies: Sexist and Racist Implications' in *Ecofeminism*, Maria Mies and Vandana Shiva, eds, Halifax, Nova Scotia: Fernwood Publications, 1993, 174–97.

————, '"Why Do We Need All This?" A Call against Genetic Engineering and Reproductive Technology', *Women's Studies International Forum* 8:6 (1985): 553–60.

Mies, Maria, and Vandana Shiva, *Ecofeminism*, Atlantic Highlands, NJ: Zed Books, 1993.

Mill, James, 'Essay on Government', (Selections) in *The Struggle for Women's Rights*, ed. George Klosko and Margaret G. Klosko, Upper Saddle River, NJ: Prentice Hall, 1999, 52–6.

Mills, Charles, *The Racial Contract*, Ithaca, NY: Cornell University Press, 1997.

Miringoff, Marque-Luisa, *The Social Costs of Genetic Welfare*, New Brunswick, NJ: Rutgers University Press, 1991.

Mitchell, Juliet, 'Women: The Longest Revolution', *New Left Review* (Nov/Dec, 1966): 40.

Mitchell, Lisa M., *Baby's First Picture: Ultrasound and the Politics of Fetal Subjects*, Toronto: University of Toronto Press, 2001.

————, 'The Routinization of the Other: Ultrasound, Women and the Fetus' in *Misconceptions: The Social Construction of Choice and the New Reproductive and Genetic Technologies*, Vol. 2, ed. Gwynne Basen, Margrit Eichler and Abby Lippman, Prescott, Ontario: Voyageur Publishing, 1994.

Moghissi, Haideh, *Feminism and Islamic Fundamentalism: The Limits of Postmodern Analysis*, New York: Zed Books, 1999.

Moller Okin, Susan, *Women in Western Political Thought*, Princeton, NJ: Princeton University Press, 1979.

Molyneux, Maxine, and Deborah Lynn Steinberg, 'Mies and Shiva's *Ecofeminism*: A New Testament?', *Feminist Review* 49 (Spring 1995): 86–107.

Molyneux, Maxine, 'Mobilization without Emancipation? Women's Interests, the State, and Revolution in Nicaragua', *Feminist Studies* 11 (Summer 1985): 227–54.

Mooney, Annabelle, and Betsy Evans, *Globalization: The Key Concepts*, London: Routledge, 2007, 76.

Moore, Pamela L., 'Selling Reproduction', in *Playing Dolly: Technocultural Formations, Fantasies, and Fictions of Assisted Reproduction*, ed. E. Ann Kaplan and Susan Squier, New Brunswick, NJ: Rutgers University Press, 1999, 80–86.

Muscati, Sina A., *Embryonic Stem Cell Research and the Law – A Canadian and International Perspective*. Honors Essay, Carleton University, Ottawa, 2002.

Nelson, Barbara, and Najma Chowdhury, eds, *Women and Politics Worldwide*, New Haven and London: Yale University Press, 1994.

Nelson, Erin, 'Case Comment: Dobson v. Dobson (Litigation Guardian)', *Health Law Review* 8:3 (Winter 1999): 30–35.

Newman, Jacquetta and Linda A. White, *Women, Politics, and Public Policy: The Political Struggles of Canadian Women*, Don Mills, Ontario: Oxford University Press, 2006.

Nicholson, Linda J., ed., *Feminism/Postmodernism*, New York: Routledge, 1990.

Nolen, Stephanie, 'Desperate Mothers Fuel India's "Baby Factories"', *The Globe and Mail*, 13 February 2009: http://www.theglobeandmail.com/news/world/desperate-mothers-fuel-indias-baby-factories/article1153508/?page=all

Nordqvist, Petra, 'Feminist Heterosexual Imaginaries of Reproduction: Lesbian Conception in Feminist Studies of Reproductive Technologies', *Feminist Theory* 9:3 (2008): 273–92.

O'Brien, Mary, 'Collective Pilgrimage: The Political Personal', *Canadian Woman Studies* 18:4 (Winter 1999): 86–91.

———, 'Feminist Theory and Dialectical Logic', in *Feminist Theory: A Critique of Ideology*, ed. Nannerl O. Keohane, Michelle Z. Rosaldo and Barbara C. Gelpi, Chicago: University of Chicago Press, 1982, 99–112.

———, *The Politics of Reproduction*, Boston: Routledge and Kegan Paul, 1981.

———, *Reproducing the World: Essays in Feminist Theory*, Boulder, CO: Westview Press, 1989.

———, 'State Power and Reproductive Freedom', *Canadian Woman Studies* 18:4 (Winter 1999): 79–85.

Oakley, Ann, *The Captured Womb: A History of the Medical Care of Pregnant Women*, Oxford: Basil Blackwell, 1986.

———, 'The History of Ultrasonography in Obstetrics', *Birth* 13 (supplement) (1986): 5–10.

Overall, Christine, Ed, *The Future of Human Reproduction*, Toronto: The Women's Press, 1989.

Palmer, Julie, 'The Placental Body in 4D: Everyday Practices of Non-Diagnostic Sonography', *Feminist Review* 93 (2009): 64–80.

———, 'Seeing and Knowing: Ultrasound Images in the Contemporary Abortion Debate', *Feminist Theory* 10 (2009): 173–89.

Paltrow, Lynn M. and Jeanne Flavin, 'Arrests of and Forced Interventions on Pregnant Women in the United States, 1973–2005: Implications for Women's Legal Status and Public Health' *Journal of Health Politics, Police and Law* (2013): 299–343.

Parpart, Jane and Marysia Zalewski, eds, *Re-Thinking the Man Question: Sex, Gender, Violence in International Relations*, London: Zed Books, 2008.

Pateman, Carole, 'The Fraternal Social Contract', in *Civil Society and the State: New European Perspectives*, ed. J. Keane, London and New York: Verso, 1988, 101–27.

———, '"God Hath Ordained to Man a Helper": Hobbes, Patriarchy and Conjugal Right', in *Feminist Interpretations and Political Theory*, ed. Mary Lyndon Shanley and Carole Pateman, University Park, PA: Pennsylvania State University Press, 1991, 53–73.

————, *The Sexual Contract*, Cambridge/Stanford: Polity/Stanford University Press, 1988.

Pearce, Tralee, 'Ending the Chore War: 5 Ideas for Peace on the Domestic Front', *The Globe and Mail*, 6 June 2013. Online.

Petchesky, Rosalind Pollack, *Abortion and Woman's Choice: The State, Sexuality and Reproductive Freedom*, Boston: Northeastern University Press, 1984.

————, 'The Body as Property: A Feminist Re-vision', in *Conceiving the New World Order: The Global Politics of Reproduction*, ed. Faye D. Ginsburg and Rayna Rapp, Berkeley: University of California, 1995, 387–406.

————, 'Foetal Images: The Power of Visual Culture in the Politics of Reproduction', in *Reproductive Technologies: Gender, Motherhood and Medicine*, ed. Michelle Stanworth, Minneapolis: University of Minnesota Press, 1987, 57–80.

————, 'Reproductive Freedom: Beyond "A Woman's Right to Choose"', *Signs – The Journal of Women in Culture and Society* 5 (Summer 1980): 661–85.

Peters, Richard S., ed., *Body, Man and Citizen: Thomas Hobbes on Logic and Methodology; Body and Motion; Sense, Animal Motion, and Human Behavior; Citizens and the Law*, New York: Collier Books, 1967.

Pfeffer, Naomi, 'Not so New Technologies', *Trouble and Strife* 5 (Spring 1985): 46–50.

————, *The Stork and the Syringe: A Political History of Reproductive Medicine*, Cambridge: Polity Press, 1993.

Phillips, Anne, *The Politics of Presence*, Oxford: Clarendon Press, 1995.

Pierce, Ellise, Julie Scelfo and Karen Springen, 'Should You Have Your Baby Now?' *Newsweek*, 13 August 2001, 40–48.

Piercy, Marge, *Woman on the Edge of Time*, New York: Ballantine Books, 1976.

Plant, Sadie, 'The Future Looms: Weaving Women and Cybernetics', in *Cybersexualities: A Reader on Feminist Theory, Cyborgs and Cyberspace*, ed. Jenny Wolmark, Edinburgh: Edinburgh University Press, 1999, 99–118.

Plato, 'The Laws', in *The Collected Dialogues of Plato*, Bollingen Series LXXI, ed. Huntington Cairns and Edith Hamilton, Princeton, NJ: Princeton University Press, 1989, 1225–513.

————, *The Republic*, trans. Richard W. Sterling and William C. Scott, New York: W.W. Norton and Company, 1985.

————, 'The Symposium', *Dialogues of Plato*, ed. J.D. Kaplan, New York: The Pocket Library, 1955.

————, *Theaetetus*, trans. John McDowell, Oxford: Clarendon Press, 1973.

Postman, Neil, *Building a Bridge to the 18th Century: How the Past Can Improve Our Future*, New York: Vintage, 2000.

Prado, C.G, *Descartes and Foucault: A Contrastive Introduction to Philosophy*, Ottawa: University of Ottawa Press, 1992.

Purdy, Laura M, 'What Can Progress in Reproductive Technology Mean for Women?' *The Journal of Medicine and Philosophy* 21:5 (1996): 499–513.

Rabinow, Paul, *Essential Works of Foucault 1954–1984*, Vol. 1, trans. Robert Hurley and Others, New York: The New Press, 1997.

Ramazanoglu, Caroline, ed., *Up Against Foucault: Explorations of Some Tensions between Foucault and Feminism*, London: Routledge, 1993.

Raymond, Janice, *Women as Wombs: Reproductive Technologies and the Battle over Women's Freedom*, San Francisco: Harper, 1993.

Rebick, Judy, 'Is the Issue Choice?', in *Misconceptions: The Social Construction of Choice and the New Reproductive and Genetic Technologies*, Vol. 1, ed. Gwynne Basen, Margrit Eichler and Abby Lippman, Prescott, Ontario: Voyageur Publishing, 1993.

Robertson, John, 'Embryos, Families, and Procreative Liberty: The Legal Structure of the New Reproduction', *Southern California Law Review* 59:5 (1986).

Rolin, Kristina, 'The Bias Paradox in Feminist Standpoint Epistemology', *Episteme: A Journal of Social Epistemology* 3:1 (2006): 125–36.

Rowland, Robyn, *Living Laboratories: Women and Reproductive Technology*, London: Lime Tree, 1992.

Rubin, Gayle, 'The Traffic in Women: Notes on the "Political Economy" of Sex', in *Toward an Anthropology of Women*, ed. Rayna Reiter, New York: Monthly Review Press, 1975.

Ruddick, Sara, 'Rethinking "Maternal" Politics', in *The Politics of Motherhood: Activist Voices from Left to Right*, ed. Alexis Jetter, Annelise Orleck, and Diana Taylor, Hanover, NH: University Press of New England, 1997, 369–81.

Sandel, Michael. Transcripts for 'Lecture 2: Morality in Politics', *BBC Reith Lectures: A New Citizenship*, 16 June 2009: http://www.bbc.co.uk/programmes/b00kt7rg

Saul, Stephanie, 'New Jersey Judge Calls Surrogate Legal Mother of Twins', *The New York Times*, 31 December 2009.

Sawicki, Jana, *Disciplining Foucault: Feminism, Power and the Body*, New York: Routledge, 1991.

———, 'Feminism, Foucault, and "Subjects" of Power and Freedom', in *Feminist Interpretations of Michel Foucault*, ed. Susan J. Hekman, University Park, PA: Pennsylvania State University Press, 1996.

———, 'Foucault, Feminism and Questions of Identity', in *The Cambridge Companion to Foucault*, ed. Gary Gutting, New York: Cambridge University Press, 1994, 286–313.

Scala, Francesca, 'Experts, Non-Experts and Policy Discourse: A Case Study of the Royal Commission on New Reproductive Technologies', PhD Diss., Carleton University, Ottawa, 2002.

Seager, Joni, *The Penguin Atlas of Women in the World*, 4th edn, New York: Penguin Books, 2009.

Seeman, Neil, 'Birth Rate Ticks, Media Roars', *Canstats Bulletins*, 12 August 2003. Accessed online 17 July 2004.

Shelley, Mary, *Frankenstein: Or the Modern Prometheus*, Ware, UK: Wordsworth Classics, 1999.

Shiva, Vandana, *Biopiracy: The Plunder of Nature and Knowledge*, Toronto: Between the Lines, 1997.

Sim, Stuart, ed., *The Routledge Critical Dictionary of Postmodern Thought*, New York: Routledge, 1999.

Singh, Navsharan, 'Contesting Reproduction; Gender, the State and Reproductive Technologies in India', PhD Diss., Carleton University, Ottawa, 1998.

Smith, Dorothy, *The Everyday World as Problematic: A Feminist Sociology*, Milton Keynes: Open University Press, 1987.

———, 'Ironies of Post-Modernism or Cheal's Doom', *Canadian Journal of Sociology* 15:3 (1990): 334–5.

Solomon, Robert C., and Kathleen M. Higgins, *A Passion for Wisdom: A Very Brief History of Philosophy*, New York: Oxford University Press, 1997.

Spallone, Patricia, *Beyond Conception: The New Politics of Reproduction*, Basingstoke: Macmillan Education Ltd, 1989.

Spar, Debora, L., *The Baby Business: How Money, Science, and Politics Drive the Commerce of Conception*, Boston: Harvard Business School Press, 2006.

Spender, Dale, *Nattering on the Net: Women, Power and Cyberspace*, Australia: Pinifex Press Pty Ltd, 1995.

———, 'The Position of Women in Information Technology – or Who Got there First and with What Consequences?', *Current Sociology* 45:2 (1997): 135–47.

Squier, Susan Merrill, *Babies in Bottles: Twentieth-Century Visions of Reproductive Technology*, New Brunswick, NJ: Rutgers University Press, 1994.

———, 'Fetal Subjects and Maternal Objects: Reproductive Technology and the New Fetal/Maternal Relation', *The Journal of Medicine and Philosophy* 21:5 (1996): 515–35.

———, *Liminal Lives: Imagining the Human at the Frontiers of Biomedicine*, Durham, NC: Duke University Press, 2004.

Stabile, Carol A., *Feminism and the Technological Fix*, Manchester: Manchester University Press, 1994.

Stanworth, Michelle, 'Birth Pangs: Conceptive Technologies and the Threat to Motherhood', in *Feminist Theory: A Reader*, ed. Wendy Kolmar and Frances Bartkowski, Mountain View, California: Mayfield Publishing Company, 1999, 454–64.

———, ed., *Reproductive Technologies: Gender, Motherhood and Medicine*, Minneapolis: University of Minnesota Press, 1987.

Stone, Alison, 'Essentialism and Anti-Essentialism in Feminist Philosophy', *Journal of Moral Philosophy* 1:2 (2004): 135–53.

Stone, Allucquere Rosanne, 'Will the Real Body Please Stand Up? Boundary Stories about Virtual Cultures', in *Cybersexualities: A Reader on Feminist Theory, Cyborgs and Cyberspace*, ed. Jenny Wolmark, Edinburgh: Edinburgh University Press, 1999, 69–98.

Strauss, Leo, *The City and the Man*, Chicago: Rand McNally, 1964.

Stryker, Susan, 'A Conversation with Susan Stryker', *International Feminist Journal of Politics* 5:1 (March 2003): 117–29.

Sunden, Jenny, 'What Happened to Difference in Cyberspace? The (Re)turn of the She-Cyborg' *Feminist Media Studies* 1:2, (2001): 215–32.

Taylor, Charles, *The Ethics of Authenticity*, Cambridge, MA: Harvard University Press, 1991.

———, *Multiculturalism and the 'Politics of Recognition'*, Princeton, NJ: Princeton University Press, 1992.

Taylor, Diana, 'Redefining Motherhood Through Technologies and Sexualities', in *The Politics of Motherhood: Activist Voices from Left to Right*, ed. Alexis Jetter, Annelise Orleck and Diana Taylor, Hanover, NH: University Press of New England, 1997, 285–7.

Thiele, Bev, 'Dissolving Dualisms: O'Brien, Embodiment and Social Construction', *Resources for Feminist Research* 18:3 (1989): 7–12.

———, 'Retrieving the Baby: Feminist Theory and Organic Bodies', *Canadian Woman Studies* 18:4 (1999): 51–9.

Thompson, Charis, *Making Parents: The Ontological Choreography of Reproductive Technologies*, USA: Massachusetts Institute of Technology Press, 2005.

Thompson, Mary, 'Third Wave Feminism and the Politics of Motherhood', *Genders OnLine Journal* 43 (2006): 10.

Thornham, Sue, 'Postmodernism and Feminism (or: Repairing our own cars)', in *The Routledge Critical Dictionary of Postmodern Thought*, ed. Stuart Sim, New York: Routledge, 1999, 41–52.

Tong, Rosemarie Putnam, *Feminist Thought: A More Comprehensive Introduction*, Boulder, CO: Westview Press, 1998.

Townley, Cynthia, *A Defense of Ignorance: Its Value for Knowers and Roles in Feminist and Social Epistemologies*, Lanham, MD: Rowman & Littlefield Publishers, 2011.

Tyler, Imogen, 'Reframing Pregnant Embodiment', in *Transformations: Thinking Through Feminism*, ed. Sara Ahmed, Janet Kilby, Celia Lury, Maureen McNeil, and Beverley Skeggs, London and New York: Routledge, 2000, 288–302.

Valverde, Mariana, and Lorna Weir, 'Regulating New Reproductive and Genetic Technologies: A Feminist View of Recent Canadian Government Initiatives', *Feminist Studies* 23:2 (Summer 1997): 419–23.

Van der Tuin, Iris and Rick Dolphijn, 'The Transversality of New Materialism', *Women: A Cultural Review* 21:2 (2010): 153–71.

Van der Tuin, Iris, 'Deflationary Logic: Response to Sara Ahmed's "Imaginary Prohibitions: Some Preliminary Remarks on the Founding Gestures of the 'New Materialism'"', *European Journal of Women's Studies* 15:4 (2008): 411–16.

———, '"Jumping Generations": On Second- and Third-wave Feminist Epistemology', *Australian Feminist Studies* 24:59 (2009): 18–31.

———, 'New Feminist Materialisms' *Women's Studies International Forum* 34 (2011): 271–77.

Vandelac, Louise, 'The Baird Commission: From "Access" to "Reproductive Technologies" to the "Excesses" of Practitioners or the Art of Diversion and

Relentless Pursuit ... ', in *Misconceptions: The Social Construction of Choice and the New Reproductive and Genetic Technologies*, Vol. 1, ed. Gwynne Basen, Margrit Eichler and Abby Lippman, Prescott, Ontario: Voyageur Publishing, 1993.

————, 'The Industrialization of Life', in *Misconceptions: The Social Construction of Choice and the New Reproductive and Genetic Technologies*, Vol. 2, ed. Gwynne Basen, Margrit Eichler and Abby Lippman, Prescott, Ontario: Voyageur Publishing, 1994, 99–114.

Vanderwater, Bette, 'Meanings and Strategies of Reproductive Control: Current Feminist Approaches to Reproductive Technology', *Issues in Reproductive and Genetic Engineering* 5:3 (1992): 215–30.

Vickers, Jill, 'Coming Up For Air: Feminist Views of Power Reconsidered', *Canadian Woman Studies* 2:4 (Winter 1980): 66–9.

————, 'Difficult Choices: The Knowledge Strategies of Feminist Social Science and the Knowledge Needs of Women's Movements', in *Quilting a New Canon: Stitching Women's Words*, ed. Uma Parameswaran, Toronto: Sister Vision, 1996, 221–40.

————, 'Notes toward a Political Theory of Sex and Power', in *Power/Gender: Social Relations in Theory and Practice*, ed. H. Lorraine Radtke and Henderikus J. Stam, London: Sage, 1994, 174–93.

————, *The Politics of 'Race': Canada, Australia, the United States*, Canada: The Golden Dog Press, 2002.

————, *Reinventing Political Science: A Feminist Approach*, Halifax, NS: Fernwood, 1997.

————, 'Whatever Happened to Sex?' *Canadian Woman Studies* 18:4 (Winter 1999).

Waring, Marilyn, *Counting for Nothing: What Men Value and What Women are Worth*, Toronto: University of Toronto Press, 1999.

Weedon, Chris, 'Postmodernism', in *A Companion to Feminist Philosophy*, ed. Alison Jaggar and Iris Marion Young, Malden, MA: Blackwell, 1998, 75–84.

Wendell, Susan, 'Feminism, Disability and Transcendence of the Body', *Canadian Woman Studies* 13:4 (Summer 1993): 117–22.

————, 'The Flight from the Rejected Body', in *Gender Basics: Feminist Perspectives on Women and Men*, ed. A. Minas, Belmont, CA: Wadsworth, 1988, 56–64.

Whitney, Shiloh Y., 'Dependency Relations: Corporeal Vulnerability and Norms of Personhood in Hobbes and Kittay', *Hypatia*, 26:3 (Summer, 2011).

Witt, Charlotte, *The Metaphysics of Gender*, New York: Oxford University Press, 2011.

Woliver, Laura R., 'The Influence of Technology on the Politics of Motherhood: An Overview of the United States', *Women's Studies International Forum* 14:5 (1991): 479–90.

Woll, Lisa, 'The Effect of Feminist Opposition to Reproductive Technology: A Case Study in Victoria, Australia', *Issues in Reproductive and Genetic Engineering* 5:1 (1992): 21–38.

Wollstonecraft, Mary, 'A Vindication of the Rights of Women', (Selections) in *The Struggle for Women's Rights: Theoretical & Historical Soucres*, ed. George Klosko and Margaret G. Klosko, Upper Saddle River, NJ: Prentice Hall, 1999, 32–51.

Wolmark, Jenny, ed., *Cybersexualities: A Reader on Feminist Theory, Cyborgs and Cyberspace*, Edinburgh: Edinburgh University Press, 1999.

Woodward, Kath and Sophie Woodward, *Why Feminism Matters: Feminism Lost and Found*, Basingstoke: Palgrave Macmillan, 2009.

Wylie, Alison, 'Why Standpoint Matters', in *Science and Other Cultures: Issues in Philosophies of Science and Technology*, ed. Robert Figueroa and Sandra Harding, New York: Routledge, 2003, 26–48.

Yeung, Miriam, 'Conceiving the Future: Reproductive-justice Activists on Technology and Policy', *Bitch: Feminist Response to Pop Culture* 40 (2008): 58–63.

Zalewski, Marysia, 'A Conversation with Susan Stryker', *International Feminist Journal of Politics* 5:1 (March 2003): 118–25.

———, *Feminism after Postmodernism: Theorising Through Practice*, London and New York: Routledge, 2000.

Index

abortion
  as choice 42, 52, 60, 62
  as consumer service 62
  embryo/foetus as rights-bearing,
    autonomous individual and 29–30
Ahmed, Sara 4 n13, 26
AIS (Androgen Insensitivity Syndrome)
  103
Alcoff, Linda 6, 13, 100, 106–7
Allucquere Stone, Rosanne 58
androcentricity: *see also* patriarchal
    dualism
  androcentic 'equality' 23
  birth appropriation and 79, 82
  continuing dominance in liberal
    societies 117, 119–20
  devaluation of woman's role and 27,
    30
  epistemic injustice and 128–9
  essentialism and 5–6
  feminist empiricism vs postmodernist
    approach to 88, 100–1
  liberal individualism and 48, 120–1,
    126–7
  NRT-based disembodiment and 15, 39,
    45, 79, 120–1, 122
  anti-natalism 8, 51–2, 54, 60, 63, 86,
    126–7
Arditti, Rita 22, 36
Arneil, Barbara 102
Asberg, Cecilia 45, 98
Atwood, Margaret (*The Handmaid's Tale*)
  44, 60
Australia, 'infertile' rights 36

Baird, Patricia 69–71
Barad, Karen 2, 92–3, 109–10, 112, 118,
  124, 126–7
Bessner, Ronda 31

biology/society dualism: *see* Cartesian
    (mind-body) dualism; dualism
    (biology/society and gender/sex);
    patriarchal dualism; trans-dualism
biosocial approach
  changing praxis and 126
  dialectical reproductive materialism
    and 2, 4–5, 12–14, 16–17, 27, 77,
    79–80, 82, 87, 94, 117
  equivocal feminists and 16, 65–6,
    75–7, 87, 113, 125
  feminist standpoint theory and 88, 90,
    94, 125
  globalization and 126
  O'Brien and 119, 122–3, 125
  policy changes resulting from 95,
    113–15, 125–6
  postconstruction/new feminine
    materialisms and 95, 113–15,
    125–6
  technoscientific progress and 126–7
Birke, Lynda 6, 7, 10–11, 13, 75, 105–6,
  114
birth appropriation
  in ancient Greece 34
  definition 3
  disembodiment and 117, 118
  as equalization of reproductive burden
    34
  NRTs, effect 3, 12–13, 33–4, 39
  patriarchal dualism and 3, 6, 8, 12,
    15–16, 34, 39–40, 42, 80, 117, 119
  patriarchal hegemony and 85
  technoscience, role 43
Brodribb, Somer 75, 83–4, 85, 86
Burfoot, Annette 9, 46, 70, 75, 84, 86,
  124–5
Butler, Judith 7, 11, 14, 43, 105–6,
  124–5

C-section as elective procedure 1, 22
Canada
    AHRA (Assisted Human Reproduction
        and Related Research Act) (2004)
        71, 125, 126
    C-section as elective procedure 1, 22
    compulsory tests on pregnant women
        51
    FINRRAGE 52, 68–9, 71
    NAC (National Action Committee on
        the Status of Women) 52, 70
    RCNRTs (Royal Commission on
        NRTs) 49, 69–72, 77
    SSFC (Social Science Federation of
        Canada) 70
capitalism: *see* globalization/capitalism
Cartesian (mind-body) dualism
    biology/society and gender/sex dualism
        and 13–14
    (dis)embodiment and 25–7, 38, 53,
        56, 81
    ongoing influence 6, 7, 8, 11, 13, 127
    patriarchal dualism and 14, 124
    postmodernism/poststructuralism and
        7, 8, 11, 95
    third wave feminism and 102
cartography methodology 80, 97, 110–12,
    118–19
choice: *see* freedom vs restriction of choice
Clarke, Adele 10–11
commodification of reproductive process
    1, 22–3, 48, 70–1, 83–4
commonality of women's experience,
    importance 6, 14, 43, 87
conceptive technology
    commodification of reproduction and
        83–4
    contraceptive technology and its
        impact distinguished 10–11, 21,
        41, 42–3, 52–3, 54, 62: *see also*
        contraceptive technology; NRTs
        (new reproductive technologies)
    devaluation of woman's role 22–3
    as disembodiment 21–3
    freedom vs restriction of choice
        consequent on 22–3, 52–3
    postmodernism and 10–11

socio-economic inequalities and 84
contraceptive technology: *see also*
    abortion; conceptive technology
    choice and 41, 84–5
    transformative nature 85
control: *see* freedom vs restriction of
    choice
Coole, Diana and Samantha Frost 109, 110
Corea, Gena 44, 48, 51, 75
cyborg/cybernetics 55, 56–9

Daniels, Cynthia 32
de Beauvoir, Simone 7–8, 51–2, 54, 60, 63
deconstruction of identity (postmodernist)
    12, 91, 100–1, 102
'dialectic' 82
dialectical reproductive materialism:
    see also Marxist dialectical
    materialism/socialist basis
    as biosocial dialect 2, 4–5, 12–14,
        27, 77, 79–80, 82, 87, 88, 94, 99,
        113–15, 117, 122–3, 125, 126
    equivocal feminists and 16, 65–6, 72,
        76, 77, 125
    feminist standpoint theory and 5–6,
        12–13, 16, 21, 74, 76, 79–80, 81,
        86–8, 90, 94
    productive vs reproductive labour
        9–10, 86
    reproductive praxis and 21
disembodiment: *see also* embodiment
    autonomy of embryo/foetus and 24,
        27–31
    birth appropriation and 117, 118
    NRTs and 1
dualism (biology/society and gender/sex)
    1–3
    biological and socio-cultural nature of
        reproductive experience 13–14
    Cartesian roots 6, 8, 14
    as perpetuation of patriarchal/
        androcentric dualism 2, 15, 67 *see*
        also patriarchal dualism

ecofeminism 21–2, 44–5
Eichler, Margrit 69–70
Eisenstein, Zillah 34, 122

embodiment: *see also* disembodiment
  as collective concept 25, 26, 120–1
  definition 25–7
  patriarchal dualism and 25, 26–7
embracing feminists and NRTs 53–60,
    61–3
  cyborg/cybernetics and 55, 56–9, 105
  essentialism and 56, 60, 61
  feminist science fiction and 53–5
  'infertile' rights 53, 56, 59–60, 61–2
  oppressive nature of reproduction and
      the body 16, 39, 53, 54, 56, 60
  patriarchal dualism and 57, 60, 61,
      66
  technophile manifesto (Firestone)
      53–5
  trans-dualism and 53–4, 60
embryo/foetus as rights-bearing,
    autonomous individual 24, 27–31
equivocal feminists and NRTs 65–77
  as biosocial/transdual response 16, 17,
      65–6, 75–7, 87, 113, 125
  dialectical reproductive materialism/
      Marxism and 16, 65–6, 72–5, 76,
      77, 125
  essentialism and 66–7, 75
  perception of the 'body' 40
  RCNRTs 49, 69–72, 77
  technophobia vs technomania 66–9
  terminology adopted by 65–6, 75–6
  trans-dualism and 16, 17, 65–6,
      76–7
essentialism
  androcentricity and 5–6
  anti-natalism/gender-focus and 8,
      66–7, 86, 105–6
  embracing feminists and 56, 60, 61
  equivocal feminists and 66–7, 75
  feminist standpoint and 89–90
  new feminisms and 98–102
  NRTs and 80
  postmodern anti-essentialism 12, 17,
      42, 60, 74–5, 80, 86, 95, 97,
      105–6
  resistance feminists and 52, 56, 61
  'situated knowledges' and 103–4
  technophobia vs technomania 66–9

universalism distinguished 5, 12, 86, 88

feminist science fiction 44–5, 53–5
feminist standpoint theory/epistemology
  biosocial dialect and 88, 90
  definition/scope of concept 81, 88
  Harding on 87–90, 93, 94, 109
  Hartsock on 5, 14, 73–4, 79–80,
      88–91, 92, 122
  individual autonomy and 26n21, 27
  multiplicity of standpoints/counter-
      hegemonic basis 5–6, 26, 73–4,
      86–7, 88–91, 115, 128–9
  O'Brien's dialectical reproductive
      materialism and 5–6, 12–13, 16,
      21, 74, 76, 79–80, 81, 86–7, 86–8,
      90, 94
  postconstructionism/new material
      feminisms and 74–5, 88
  postmodernism/poststructuralism and
      91, 92
  reproductive consciousness and 12
  socialist/Marxist basis 73–5, 88–90,
      92–3, 94, 95
  uniqueness of women's perspectives as
      core 74
feminist waves: *see also* linear/teleological
    approach, difficulties with;
    postconstructionism/new
    material feminisms, 'new',
    'renewed' or parallel?
  breaking feminist waves 100, 106–8
  modern second wave/postmodern
      third wave antagonism 4, 99–100,
      106–7
  'third wave' defined 102n27
  third wave/post-natural body 102–3
  trans-dualistic/'postdisciplinary
      famework' and 107–8
Firestone, Shulamith 8, 16, 34, 41, 42,
    53–5, 59, 60, 61, 63, 66–7
foetomaternal microchimerism 126–7
freedom vs restriction of choice
  abortion and 42, 52, 60, 62
  conceptive and contraceptive
      technology distinguished 41,
      52–3, 62

disabilities, relevance 7, 14–15, 35–6,
    41, 51, 53, 57–8, 59–60, 61–2,
    68–9, 121–4
  individual and collective choice
    distinguished 42–3, 48–9, 52–3,
    61, 62, 65–6, 70–1, 76–7, 84
  as market concept 62
  NRTs and 1, 9, 13–14, 21–3, 35, 38,
    41–63
  obligatory pregnancy tests 51
  patriarchal dualism and 60, 61
  patriarchal hegemony and 1, 34, 50–1,
    52–3
  resistance feminists' approach 42–3,
    48–53, 61–3
  rights distinguished 62
  socio-economic considerations 32–3,
    50–2, 61, 62, 67, 68–9
  technological progress as priority and
    50–1
Friedan, Betty 107

Garland-Thomson, Rosemarie 13–14,
    74n44, 98–9, 117, 121, 122–4,
    128–9
gays: *see* lesbians, gays, transsexuals/
    transgendered and the effect of
    NRTs
geneticization of health and reproduction
    1, 50, 126
globalization/capitalism
  biosocial approach and 126
  biotechnology revolution and 21,
    126
  postmodernism and 8–10
  as source of patriarchal oppression 51,
    56–7, 72–3, 83–4, 89, 128–9
Grant, Judit 3n10
Greer, Germaine 16, 42, 43, 46, 103

Hadd, Wendi 26–7, 29, 38
Haraway, Donna 53, 56–7, 58, 66,
    74n44, 90–2, 99, 103–6, 128
Harding, Sandra 73, 75n46, 87–8, 89–90,
    93, 94, 109
Hartouni, Valerie 24, 30, 48
Hartsock, Nancy

feminist standpoint theory 5, 14,
    73–4, 79–80, 88–91, 92, 122: *see
    also* feminist standpoint theory/
    epistemology
  on Haraway 103
  on O'Brien 86, 87
Hekman, Susan and Stacy Alaimo 98–9,
    106
hermeneutic approach, importance 7, 75,
    90
Howie, Gillian 5, 6, 75, 98–9, 100, 106–7,
    108, 128

infertility/'infertile' rights: *see also*
    lesbians, gays, transsexuals/
    transgendered and the effect of
    NRTs
  Australia 36
  ecofeminism and 44–5
  globalized capitalism and 9
  NRTs as solution? 9–10, 35–6, 43,
    48–53
  psychological infertility 36
  RCNRTs and 49
  resistance feminists' approach to
    48–53
  sociological solutions 50
  UK 67
  US 36, 67
  variable/socio-cultural concept 48–52
IVF (*in vitro* fertilization)
  'choice' and 51
  devaluation of woman's role 31
  disembodiment and 1, 27
  Louise Brown (1978) 31
  radical vs socialist feminist split 75
  socio-economic class and 67, 72
  UK 75

James, P.D. 44
Jameson, Frederic 9–10
Johnson, Candace 37, 68

Katz-Rothman, Barbara 50–1
Kruks, Sonia 92–3

Legge M., R. Fitzgerald and N. Frank 36–7

lesbians, gays, transsexuals/transgendered
    and the effect of NRTs
    AIS (Androgen Insensitivity
        Syndrome) 103
    embracing feminists and 53, 56,
        59–60, 61–2
    entitlement to fertility services 35–7,
        68–9, 72
    equivocal feminists and 72
    gender categorizations 102–3
    reproductive justice and 63
    as transformative change 41
Lie, Merete 46, 49
linear/teleological approach, difficulties
        with 73n40, 75n46, 94, 100, 109:
        see also feminist waves
    cartography alternative 80, 97,
        110–12, 118–19
Lippman, Abby 22, 50
Lublin, Nancy 25, 54–5, 66–7, 69, 75–6
Lykke, Nina 2–3, 80, 87–8, 90–1, 93,
        94, 99, 100, 103, 105, 107, 109,
        111, 123
Lynn M. Paltrow and Jeanne Flavin 31–2

Makus, Ingrid 22–3
Marxist dialectical materialism/socialist
        basis: *see also* dialectical
        reproductive materialism
    cross-feminist waves and 108
    feminist standpoint and 73–5, 88–90,
        92–3, 94, 95
    Hartsock and 88–9
    O'Brien and 11–12, 81–7
    postconstructionism/new material
        feminisms and 94, 95, 109–10
    postmodern/Marxist materialism
        tensions 93, 95
    productive vs reproductive labour
        9–10, 86
    socialist feminism and 72–4
material feminisms: *see*
        postconstructionism/new material
        feminisms
Matthews, Gwyneth 59–60
Menzies, Heather 65
Merchant, Carolyn 21–2, 44–5, 56
Mies, Maria 44, 49

misfitting 74, 88, 117, 121–4
Mitchell, Juliet 73, 92
Mitchell, Lisa 25, 27, 28n26, 29, 47

new material feminisms: *see*
        postconstructionism/new material
        feminisms
NRTs (new reproductive technologies):
        see also conceptive technology
    alternative terminology 24–5
    commodification of reproductive
        process and 1, 22–3, 29, 48, 70–1,
        83–4
    devaluation of woman's role 30–1
    embracing feminists and: *see*
        embracing feminists and NRTs
    equivocal feminists and: *see* equivocal
        feminists and NRTs
    examples 1
    as expression of postmodernism 1, 3,
        9–10, 13
    Firestone on 54–5
    globalization and 9, 21
    patriarchal hegemony and 52–3
    reproductive consciousness and 22–3,
        75, 83–4, 118
    resistance feminists and: *see* resistance
        feminists and NRTs
    transformative nature 9, 21–2, 23, 25

O'Brien, Mary: *see also* dialectical
        reproductive materialism;
        reproductive consciousness
    biological essentialist/social
        constructionist divide and 2, 4–7,
        12, 13–14, 75, 90, 117
    biosocial reproduction
        embodiment/agent of creation and
            27, 34, 76
        patriarchal nature/culture dualism
            and 16–17, 79, 127
    commodification of women 22
    contraceptive technology as working
        environment 21
    Marxism and 11–12, 81–7
    materialist theory of reproduction
        4–5, 121

feminist standpoint epistemology
    and 80–7, 91, 94
new material feminisms and 76, 79,
    80, 122–3
NRTs, attitude to 13
'world historically significant'
    moments of change 3, 4, 12,
    118–19
Our Bodies Ourselves (Boston Health
    Collective) 26, 45

Palmer, Julie 24n15, 28, 29
paternity as physiological concept 3, 21,
    84–5, 118
patriarchal dualism: *see also*
    androcentricity; dualism (biology/
    society and gender/sex); trans-
    dualism
birth appropriation 3, 6, 8, 12, 15–16,
    34, 39–40, 42, 80, 117, 119
Cartesian dualism and 14
choice and 60, 61
embracing feminists and 57, 60, 61, 66
'equivocal' feminist response to 16,
    65–6, 75–7, 125
examples 2
feminist strategies and 13
man/technology–woman/nature binary
    16, 21–2, 39–40, 42, 44–7, 57, 61,
    65
postmodernism and 8
resistance feminists and 42, 43–7,
    61
transformative role of NRTs 21–2
patriarchal hegemony
birth appropriation and 85
freedom vs restriction of choice 1, 34,
    50–1, 52–3
NRTs and 52–3
uncertainty of paternity and 85
Petchesky, Rosalind 29, 47, 67, 68, 76
Pfeffer, Naomi 68–9
Piercy, Marge 53–4, 55
Plant, Sadie 57, 58–9
postconstructionism/new material
    feminisms
as biosocial framework for policy-
    making 95, 113–15, 125–6

breaking feminist waves methodology
    and 110–13, 114
corpomaterialism and 93
definition 2–3
interchangeability of concepts 2–3
mediation of postmodernism/
    modernism impasse 73, 108,
    110–11, 113, 114
'new', 'renewed' or parallel? 109–13
    Barad 109–10, 112
    Burfoot 124–5
    Colebrook 110
    Coole and Frost 109
    Derrida 110
    Haraway 2–3
    Lykke 109, 111–12, 123
    Van der Tuin and Dolphijn 110–13
postmodern/Marxist materialism
    tensions and 93, 95
as a thinking technology (Haraway)
    2–3, 16–17, 79, 80, 99, 125
postmodernism/poststructuralism
androcentricity and 88, 100–1, 127
anti-essentialism 12, 17, 42, 60, 74–5,
    80, 86, 95, 97, 105–6
cyborg/cybernetics and 55, 56–9, 105
deconstruction of identity 12, 91,
    100–1, 102
definition and scope 8–9
equivalence of terms 3n10
feminist standpoint epistemology and
    91, 92
globalization and 8–9
modern/postmodern antagonism 4,
    73, 97, 99–102, 104, 106–7, 108,
    110–11, 114
    new material feminisms as means
        of mediation 73, 108, 110–11,
        113, 114
modern/postmodern timeline 10
NRTs as expression of 1, 3, 9–10, 13
patriarchal/Cartesian dualism and 7,
    8, 11, 95
postmodern/Marxist materialism
    tensions 93, 95
psychoanalysis and 73, 84, 92, 108
poststructuralism: *see* postmodernism/
    poststructuralism

praxis (reproductive, political and
    patriarchal), significance of
    changes in 3–4, 6, 8–11, 21, 23,
    75–6, 80, 82–3, 117
prostitution 48, 83

Raymond, Janice 33, 50, 52
Rebick, Judy 51, 61
reproductive consciousness
    biosocial basis 87, 90
    feminist historical materialism and
        79–80
    feminist standpoint theory/
        epistemology and 12
    masculine reproductive consciousness
        12–13
    masculinization of women's
        reproductive consciousness 33–4,
        39, 46, 118
    maternity as basis for 85
    NRTs and 22–3, 75, 83–4, 118
    as over-fragmentation 41
    patriarchal dualism and 12–14, 15, 39,
        80, 83–4, 87
    sex/gender dialect and 5, 41
    as universal vs differentiated
        experience 4, 5–6
reproductive justice 63, 76
reproductive tourism 23, 48, 126
resistance feminists and NRTs 42–53
    commonality of women's experience
        and 43
    ecofeminism and 44–5
    feminist science fiction and 44–5
    FINRRAGE 52, 68–9, 71
    freedom vs restriction of choice and
        42–3, 48–53, 61–3
    infertility and 48–53
    oppressive nature of reproduction/the
        body 39, 51–2
    patriarchal dualism and 42, 43–7, 61
Rose, Hilary 68
Rowland, Robyn 43, 50, 52

Shiva, Vandana 16, 42, 44
situated knowledges 2, 11n36, 66, 75,
    81, 88, 90–1, 99, 103–5, 118, 119,
    120

Spallone, Patricia 44n11, 45–6, 47, 50,
    51n45, 52, 75
Squier, Susan 27–9, 47, 48
Stabile, Carol 65–6, 67, 75–7
Stanworth, Michelle 30–1, 68, 72, 75
Stryker, Susan 56, 102–3
surrogacy
    AHRA ban on paid arrangements 126
    Baby M case (1988) 32–3
    cross-class surrogacy 23, 48
    devaluation of surrogate mother's role
        22, 30–1
    disaggregation of reproduction 1
    genetic vs gestational ('pure')
        surrogacy 22, 32–4, 86, 127
    The Handmaid's Tale (Atwood) 44
    Johnson v. Calvert (1990) 22, 33–4,
        127
    reproductive tourism 23, 48, 126

Taylor, Charles 26
Taylor, Diana 32, 35
technoscience as [male-oriented]
    reconfiguration of the parameters
    1, 10–11, 42–3, 45–7, 49–50, 56,
    126–7
teleological approach: *see* linear/
    teleological approach, difficulties
    with
a thinking technology (Haraway) 2–3,
    16–17, 79, 80, 99, 125
trans-dualism
    breaking feminist waves 107
    cartography/transversal approach and
        111, 114–15
    embracing feminists and 53–4, 60
    equivocal feminists and 16, 17, 65–6,
        76–7
    new material feminisms/
        postconstructionism and 2–3,
        16–17, 66, 79, 80, 109–10
    scope 6–7
transsexuals/transgendered: *see* lesbians,
    gays, transsexuals/transgendered
    and the effect of NRTs
Tyler, Imogen 27

ultrasound imaging 24, 27–30, 47, 51

United Kingdom
    'infertile' rights 67
    IVF treatment 75
United States
    compulsory testing of pregnant
        women 29
    infertile' rights 36

Van der Tuin, Iris 73n40, 80, 93–4, 98, 99
Van der Tuin, Iris and Rick Dolphijn 95,
        97, 109, 110–13, 114–15

Wendell, Susan 37, 38, 59, 63, 124
Woliver, Laura 31
Woodward, Kath and Sophie Woodward
        5, 6, 11, 26, 74, 98, 99, 100n16,
        106, 107

Zalewski, Marysia 6, 73, 92, 100–1, 106,
        107, 108